THE LIVING HEART GUIDE TO EATING OUT

Second Edition

MICHAEL E. DeBAKEY, MD
ANTONIO M. GOTTO, JR., MD, DPhil
LYNNE W. SCOTT, MA, RD, LD

THE LIVING HEART GUIDE TO EATING OUT

Second Edition

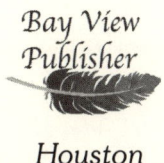

Bay View Publisher

Houston

First Edition copyright © 1993, Second Edition copyright © 2005, Michael E. DeBakey, Antonio M. Gotto, Jr., and Lynne W. Scott.

All rights reserved, including the right of reproduction in whole or in part in any form.
Published by BayView Publisher

Designed by C K Productions
Manufactured in the United States of America
10 9 8 7 6 5 4 3 2

For information call 713-794-0240 or visit www.LivingHeart.com

CONTENTS

Acknowledgment, vii
Preface, ix

1 LOWERING CHOLESTEROL AND EATING OUT—IS IT POSSIBLE TO DO BOTH? 1

High Cholesterol Is a Major Risk Factor for Heart Disease 1
What Causes High Cholesterol? 2
How to Lower Your Cholesterol 2
Dietary Choices to Lower Cholesterol 3
Determine Your Saturated Fat Allowance 4
Include Favorite Foods 5
Before You Eat Out 5
Finding Fat and Sodium in Restaurant Foods 6
Special Requests 8

2 AMERICAN CUISINE 11

Breakfast and Brunch 11
Lunch and Dinner 16
Appetizers and Soups 18
Salads and Salad Bars 20
Entrées 23
Sandwiches 26
Pizza 30
Vegetables 31
Breads and Crackers 34
Desserts 35
Beverages 37
Snacks 40

3 ETHNIC CUISINES 43

Cajun and Creole Cuisine 44
Chinese Cuisine 48
French Cuisine 52
Greek Cuisine 56
Indian Cuisine 60
Italian Cuisine 64

Japanese Cuisine *68*
Mexican Cuisine *72*
Thai Cuisine *77*
Vietnamese Cuisine *80*

4 FAST FOOD *83*

Arby's *84*
Burger King *88*
Chick-fil-A *91*
Dairy Queen *94*
Domino's Pizza *97*
Dunkin' Donuts *101*
Einstein Bros Bagels *104*
Fazoli's Italian Restaurants *107*
Jamba Juice *110*
Kentucky Fried Chicken *112*
Krispy Kreme Doughnuts *114*
Long John Silver's *115*
McDonald's *117*
Panda Express *121*
Pizza Hut *122*
Smoothie King *126*
Starbucks *128*
Subway *134*
Taco Bell *138*

5 TRAVELING *143*

Airline and Cruise Ship Cuisine *143*
Jet Lag *143*
Gastrointestional Upset in Foreign Countries *144*

About the Authors *146*
Order Forms *149*

ACKNOWLEDGEMENT

It was a pleasure working on the second edition of THE LIVING HEART GUIDE TO EATING OUT with Frances B. Hannsz. We are grateful to her for tabulating values from the extensive, latest data on fast foods. We appreciate receiving permission to use the Nutrition Data System for research software version 4.06 developed by the Nutrition Coordinating Center, University of Minnesota, MN, Food and Nutrient Database 34, released May 2003, for determining nutrient values for the American and ethnic foods. The authors are grateful to the staff in Publications & Creative Services at Baylor College of Medicine in Houston, Texas, for their assistance in the production of this book.

PREFACE

The *Living Heart* series of books spans four decades and includes *The Living Heart* and the New York Times Best Seller *The Living Heart Diet*. The initial edition of *The Living Heart Guide to Eating Out* when published in 1993 was among the first—and was perhaps the first—companion book for those who wish to continue a heart-healthy lifestyle when eating away from home. Today the guide remains the leader because its recommendations are based on both clinical experience and the latest research findings rather than on fad or personal interest. It provides simple, factual help in a time when there is truly a plethora of dietary recommendations. In many ways, a stalwart heart is needed to have a healthy heart.

This 2005, updated edition increasingly emphasizes lowering blood cholesterol, arguably the primary risk factor for a heart attack, by decreasing saturated fat intake. Decreasing saturated fat in the diet is the most powerful lifestyle change for reducing risk for a heart attack. In the chapters on typical "American" and ethnic cuisines and fast foods, values for calories, fat, and saturated fat are updated, and carbohydrate values are provided. The values often reflect larger serving sizes than were presented in the original edition of the book. Today, the average restaurant salad plate is the size of what used to be considered a dinner plate, and dinner plates are often the size of serving dishes. Carbohydrate values have been added to show interested readers where carbohydrate is in restaurant foods, including fast foods. The chapter on fast foods, completely revised, adds several restaurants.

The related website is **www.livingheart.com**. It provides more detailed guidance for readers who wish to receive a personalized diet with a meal plan and menus at the calorie level needed to lose or to maintain weight. The website's Nutrient Analyzer gives immediate feedback on calories, fat, saturated fat, carbohydrate, and 13 other nutrients in foods entered into it. Please feel free to contact us there, and we hope that this book contributes to better health and more enjoyable eating out for people of all ages.

—The Authors

CHAPTER 1

LOWERING CHOLESTEROL AND EATING OUT—IS IT POSSIBLE TO DO BOTH?

High cholesterol is dangerous. It is a major risk factor for heart disease, which will develop in one of every two men and one of every three women during their lifetime. Whether you already have heart disease or want to prevent it, you can reduce your risk for having a heart attack by lowering your blood cholesterol.

HIGH CHOLESTEROL IS A MAJOR RISK FACTOR FOR HEART DISEASE

The higher your blood cholesterol, the greater your risk for having a heart attack. Heart disease is the number one killer of men and women in the USA. Each year, more than a million Americans will have a heart attack and about half a million people will die of heart disease. *High cholesterol does NOT cause symptoms.*

Know Your Cholesterol

Everyone 20 years of age or older should know his or her cholesterol value. If it is not at a desirable level, talk with your physician.

Cholesterol	**Desirable**
Total cholesterol	Less than 200 mg/dL
LDL-cholesterol ("bad" cholesterol)	Less than 100 mg/dL
HDL-cholesterol ("good" cholesterol)	Higher than 60 mg/dL
TC:HDL ratio	Less than 4.5
LDL:HDL ratio	Less than 3

Note: Ratios are obtained by dividing TC (total cholesterol) by HDL-cholesterol and by dividing LDL-cholesterol by HDL-cholesterol.

Elevated triglycerides can also increase risk for heart disease. The desirable level of triglycerides in the blood is 150 mg/dL or lower.

WHAT CAUSES HIGH CHOLESTEROL?

Several factors you can control and others you cannot control affect your blood cholesterol level.

Factors You CAN Control: Lifestyle

Diet: A diet high in saturated fat, trans fat, and dietary cholesterol raises blood cholesterol. Foods high in saturated fat, trans fat, and cholesterol are listed on page 3.

Weight: Being overweight is a risk factor for heart disease and may increase your blood cholesterol. Losing weight helps lower your cholesterol as well as your triglycerides. Losing weight also helps increase HDL ("good") cholesterol.

Physical Activity: Being inactive is a risk factor for heart disease. Regular physical activity helps lower cholesterol, decrease triglycerides, and raise HDL-cholesterol.

Factors You CANNOT Control

Age and Gender: Cholesterol increases with age. Before menopause, women have lower total cholesterol than men of the same age. After menopause, women's LDL-cholesterol tends to rise.

Heredity: High cholesterol runs in families. While your genes partly determine your cholesterol, your diet plays a key role.

To calculate your risk for having a heart attack, visit www.livingheart.com

Lowering your cholesterol is a critical first step toward reducing your risk for heart disease.

HOW TO LOWER YOUR CHOLESTEROL

There are two proven ways to lower cholesterol:

Diet and Lifestyle Changes: A diet low in saturated fat, trans fat, and cholesterol, along with regular physical activity and weight loss (if overweight), will lower blood cholesterol and reduce your chance of developing heart disease. The addition of soluble fiber and plant stanols/sterols also helps lower blood cholesterol. Plant stanols/sterols are in specially formulated foods, such as margarines.

Medication: For some people it is necessary to add medication to lifestyle changes to decrease cholesterol to the goal level. If your physician prescribes cholesterol-lowering medication, it is important to take it daily as prescribed. *If medication is needed, it is in addition to diet, not in place of it.*

DIETARY CHOICES TO LOWER CHOLESTEROL

Decrease saturated fat to less than 7 percent of calories. Decreasing saturated fat is the most effective way to lower blood cholesterol. The major sources are:
- High-fat dairy—butter, whole milk, cheese, cream, and ice cream
- High-fat meats—fatty beef, pork, and lamb, as well as poultry skin and lard
- Tropical oils—palm oil, coconut oil, and palm kernel oil

Limit trans fat. The major sources are:
- Foods prepared with hydrogenated oils—shortening and stick margarine—and partially hydrogenated oils
- Commercially baked and fried foods—French fries, fried meat, doughnuts, crackers, cookies, regular microwave popcorn, and popcorn popped in movie theaters

Limit dietary cholesterol to less than 200 mg per day. It is only in foods of animal origin:
- Egg yolk (2 per week)
- Meat, whether lean or fatty
- Dairy products

Lose weight if you are overweight.
- To lose 1 to 2 pounds per week, decrease calories by 500 to 1000 per day.

Exercise regularly.
- At least 30 minutes a day is usually recommended. Check with your physician before starting an exercise program.

Increase soluble fiber through certain:
- Cereal grains—barley, oatmeal, oat bran, and psyllium seeds
- Fruit —apples, bananas, blackberries, citrus fruit (orange and grapefruit), pears, and prunes
- Legumes—beans, lentils, and peas
- Vegetables—Brussels sprouts and carrots

DETERMINE YOUR SATURATED FAT ALLOWANCE

Limiting saturated fat to less than 7 percent of your calories means limiting the number of grams of saturated fat in foods eaten. To determine your goals for maximum calories and grams of saturated fat daily, use 4 easy steps:

1. Rate your activity level.
   - 12 = Very little activity
   - 13 = Inactive (sedentary office worker)
   - 14 = Slightly inactive (occasional walks)
   - 15 = Moderately active (jogging, tennis, or regular calisthenics)
   - 16 = Highly active (almost always on the go)
2. Multiply your current weight by your activity level (from #1).
   Example: for a 160-pound person who has very little activity, 160 x 12 = 1920 calories
3. To lose 1 to 2 pounds per week, subtract 500 to 1000 calories per day.
   Example: 1920 − 500 = 1420 calories
4. Find your calorie level in the table below to find your recommended maximum daily amount of saturated fat.
   Example: 1400 calories = 11 grams saturated fat

Calories	Grams of Saturated Fat Equal to 7 Percent of Calories
1200	9
1400	11
1600	12
1800	14
2000	16
2200	17
2400	18
2600	20
2800	22
3000	23

Knowing how to choose foods low in saturated fat makes it easier to stay on a cholesterol-lowering diet.

INCLUDE FAVORITE FOODS

By using the previous table to estimate your saturated fat allowance, you can plan meals in restaurants and fast food places to include some of your favorite choices and stay within your allowance of saturated fat. For example, at the 2000-calorie level, with 16 grams of saturated fat, lasagna with meat, which has 15 grams saturated fat, can be worked into your diet. To include lasagna for your evening meal, select:

- Breakfast foods without saturated fat, such as cereal with skim milk and fruit
- Lunch foods that are very low in saturated fat, such as a soup and salad bar; select vegetable soup, salad with lots of vegetables, low-fat or fat-free salad dressing, melba toast, and fruit for dessert
- Dinner foods to accompany lasagna, such as minestrone soup, Italian bread dipped in olive oil, and melon for dessert

Tips for foods low in saturated fat are given in each of the Chapters on American, ethnic, and fast foods.

Substitute unsaturated fat for saturated fat. When eating out, request:

- Olive oil for salad instead of creamy dressing
- Olive or canola oil be used to baste grilled fish and meat
- Avocado to go with salad instead of dressing
- Soft tub margarine instead of butter or stick margarine

BEFORE YOU EAT OUT

There are a number of things to consider in making dining out an enjoyable heart-healthy experience. The first is what you say to yourself about eating out. You may find yourself choosing foods high in fat and saturated fat and using the excuse that "this is a special occasion" or "it can't hurt to eat foods with a lot of cheese once in a while." If you eat lunch out five days out of seven and dine out in the evening several times each week, eating out may be a major contributor to your intake of fat and saturated fat. Another common thought is that "cleaning your plate is getting your money's worth"; however, it is poor finances to eat more than you want or need.

- Plan ahead. Choose foods low in fat and saturated fat for other meals and snacks when you are going to eat out, to compensate for higher levels in restaurant foods.
- Don't skip meals in anticipation of eating out; you will be hungrier and more likely to overeat.
- Choose a place to eat that offers a wide variety of foods. Table-service restaurants with a varied menu give more choices than specialty establishments with limited menus, such as steakhouses and pizza places.

FINDING FAT AND SODIUM IN RESTAURANT FOODS

Many foods high in fat are also high in saturated fat; selecting foods low in fat will help you have less saturated fat. Fat in food can be either visible or invisible. Invisible fat is found in fatty meats (prime rib, hamburger meat, sausage, and luncheon meats), poultry skin, whole milk, cream, cheese, and desserts (pie, cake, cookies, and ice cream). Sources of visible fat include margarine, butter, oil, mayonnaise, and salad dressings. Fried foods and commercial baked goods are common sources of trans fat and should be avoided to help lower blood cholesterol.

MENU TERMS INDICATING LITTLE OR NO FAT USED IN FOOD PREPARATION

- Baked (without added fat)
- Broiled (without added fat)
- Grilled
- Poached
- Roasted
- Steamed
- Tomato sauce

> **MENU TERMS INDICATING
> A FOOD HIGH IN FAT
> AND SATURATED FAT**
>
> - Au gratin
> - Basted
> - Braised
> - Buttered/butter sauce/buttery
> - Casserole
> - Cheese sauce
> - Creamed/cream sauce/creamy
> - Crispy
> - Escalloped/scalloped
> - Fried/deep-fried
> - Gravy/in its own gravy
> - Hash
> - Hollandaise
> - Pan-fried
> - Parmesan
> - Potpie
> - Prime (the grade of meat with the most fat)
> - Sautéed
> - Stuffed

Sodium

Restaurant foods that are low in fat are not necessarily low in sodium; for example, lean ham and dill pickles are both high in sodium. Foods can be high in sodium from the sodium present in ingredients, such as cheese, sausage, and soy sauce, or from salt added in food preparation. The American and ethnic restaurant food tables in this book do not include values for sodium because preciseness is impossible. Some chefs add a generous amount of salt and others use it sparingly.

> **MENU TERMS INDICATING A FOOD HIGH IN SODIUM**
>
> - Broth or au jus (although these terms can mean served with juices from cooking, many restaurants use a prepared meat base that is high in sodium)
> - Cocktail sauce
> - Pickled
> - Smoked
> - Soy sauce and teriyaki sauce
> - Tomato base

SPECIAL REQUESTS

Most chefs want to please their customers and are usually willing to make requested changes in menu items to ensure that customers enjoy their meal. Many chefs will make the following changes:

- Serve sauce and salad dressing on the side.
- Prepare foods with vegetable oil or margarine instead of butter, lard, or shortening.
- Broil or bake an entrée rather than fry it.
- Remove the skin on chicken before cooking.
- Cook without salt.

Some foods cannot be changed upon request because they are prepared ahead of time. Examples include soups, sauces, casseroles, cornbread, crêpe fillings, and baked desserts. Fortunately, many foods can be changed, primarily those that are cooked at the time they are ordered.

However, many customers are reluctant to request menu substitutions or to make special requests about food preparation. Calling ahead to the restaurant gives these customers an excellent opportunity to ask the chef or maitre d' which foods are low in fat, whether the restaurant can accommodate special requests, and what ingredients are present in specific foods. (The best time to call most restaurants is between 3:30 and 5:30 p.m.) Here are some sample questions you may wish to ask about restaurant food, either when calling ahead or when ordering:

- Which menu items can be modified to reduce fat and/or sodium?
- Is the fat trimmed off before meat is cooked?
- Is the skin removed before chicken is cooked?
- What type of fat (if any) is used in cooking a specific entrée?
- Does a particular entrée include sauce or gravy?
- Are the cooked vegetables seasoned with butter?
- Which sauces have the least amount of fat?
- Is butter or margarine served at the table? If butter, can soft tub margarine be requested?

You may find it useful to obtain a copy of the menu before you visit a restaurant. Most restaurants have fax machines and can provide a copy of their menu immediately. Access to the menu allows you to study the dishes being offered and consider the options available.

> It is important to remember that, as the paying customer, you should not be afraid to ask for exactly what you want, and you should expect to get it—you deserve the best!

CHAPTER 2

AMERICAN CUISINE

The cuisine in the United States is a rich mixture of sources and traditions. Nearly all the dishes typically served in American restaurants are adoptions or adaptions, whether recent or of long standing. Apple pie, for instance, was a favorite dessert during the reign of Elizabeth I of England, as well as in colonial America. American Indians toasted popcorn long beforre the arrival of European explorers, and pizza as we know it, made with tomatoes, appears to have originated in Naples in the 1500s. Creole gumbo combines African, American Indian, and European elements and is an example of the regional variations of American cuisine. This chapter provides estimates of the calories, fat, saturated fat, and carbohydrate in popular American foods eaten at breakfast and brunch and for lunch and dinner. The chapter on fast food (which is very American) begins on page 83.

BREAKFAST AND BRUNCH

Food eaten at breakfast can be an important contribution to your day's food intake. If you eat lunch or dinner away from home on a regular basis, consider compensating for the saturated fat in restaurant food by making breakfast an almost fat-free meal. It is easy to do, even when you are eating out, as shown in the next table.

TIPS ON ORDERING LOWER-FAT FOOD AT BREAKFAST OR BRUNCH

- Ask for low-fat or skim milk as a beverage, for cereal, and in coffee (instead of cream).
- Request that butter or margarine not be added to grits or cooked cereals.
- Select dry cereal rather than granola, which is usually high in fat.

(continued)

TIPS ON ORDERING LOWER-FAT FOOD AT BREAKFAST OR BRUNCH *(continued)*

- Order toast, English muffins, or bagels "dry," with margarine served on the side. Then use a small amount of margarine at the table. It will probably be less than would have been added in the kitchen. Waiting until the bread cools slightly before adding margarine decreases the amount that is absorbed. Or skip the margarine and use jam or jelly instead.
- Order pancakes or waffles with fruit topping, syrup, or yogurt topping. If you use margarine, have it served on the side so that you can control the amount used.
- Order a plain poached, a soft-cooked, or a hard-cooked egg (within the recommended limit of 2 egg yolks per week).
- Request that egg substitute or egg whites be used for omelets and scrambled eggs; regular omelets often contain two to three whole eggs. Ask the chef to prepare an egg white and mushroom omelet or a Spanish omelet without cheese and served with salsa.
- Select toast and lean ham instead of breakfast sandwiches, which are usually high in calories, fat, and saturated fat because they contain a biscuit or croissant, sausage or bacon, cheese, refried beans, and/or eggs.
- If you have meat, select lean ham, Canadian bacon, or a breakfast steak instead of bacon or sausage, and count it as part of your meat intake for the day.

TIPS ON LOWERING SODIUM

- Select fruit or fruit juice instead of tomato or vegetable juice, which are high in sodium.
- Skip meat at breakfast, because even lower-fat choices, such as Canadian bacon and lean ham, are high in sodium.
- When ordering an omelet (as part of your egg allowance), ask that salt and cheese be omitted.

The following table gives you an idea of the calories, fat, saturated fat, and carbohydrate content of selected breakfast and brunch foods. The values are estimates; the content of an actual dish may vary, depending on how the chef prepares it.

	Calories	Fat g	Sat. Fat g	Carb. g
FRUIT AND JUICE				
Apple juice (1 c)	136	0	0	34
Banana (1)	108	1	0	28
Cantaloupe (½ med)	97	1	0	23
Grapefruit (½)	42	0	0	11
Grapefruit juice (1 c)	115	0	0	28
Orange juice (1 c)	105	0	0	25
Strawberry slices (½ c)	25	0	0	6
EGG DISHES AND CRÊPES				
Crêpes, chicken (2) w/cream sauce	728	24	19	56
Egg, poached, no fat added (1)	77	5	2	1
Egg, scrambled, w/butter (2)	221	17	7	3
Egg, soft-boiled, no fat added (1)	77	5	2	1
Eggs Benedict (2 eggs, 1 English muffin, 3 oz ham, hollandaise sauce)	718	46	21	36
Omelet, plain (3 eggs)	385	33	8	2
Cheese	544	46	17	3
Ham & cheese	652	54	27	2
Spanish	516	35	16	30

	Calories	Fat g	Sat. Fat g	Carb. g
Quiche (⅙ of 9")				
w/bacon	466	34	15	22
w/mushroom	403	28	13	22
w/seafood	413	28	13	21
w/spinach	405	28	13	23

BAKED GOODS

	Calories	Fat g	Sat. Fat g	Carb. g
Bagel, plain (5 oz)	390	2	0	76
Banana bread (1 sl)	122	5	1	19
Biscuit, buttermilk (2)	186	8	2	25
Cinnamon roll w/fruit, nuts & frosting (4½" x 3")	454	19	8	66
Coffeecake, w/streusel topping (3" x 3" x 1½")	468	23	6	60
Croissant (1 lg)	305	18	11	31
Danish pastry (4½" diam)				
w/cheese filling & frosting	494	27	14	55
w/fruit filling & frosting	547	25	13	76
Doughnut (4" diam)				
Plain cake w/sugar	247	13	3	28
Yeast, glazed	412	22	8	49
w/nuts, coconut & frosting	439	23	8	52
w/creme filling	397	22	8	45
English muffin, toasted, dry (1)	134	1	0	26
French toast (2 lg)	290	12	3	33
Muffin (3½" diam)				
Apple or blueberry w/ streusel topping	556	24	10	78
Bran w/streusel topping	556	24	10	78
Chocolate chip	491	20	7	70
Oat bran w/streusel topping	621	29	11	80
Raisin toast, dry (1 sl)	88	1	0	17
Scone (1 sm, 2 oz)	246	10	3	34
White or whole-wheat toast, dry (1 sl)	80	1	0	15

	Calories	Fat g	Sat. Fat g	Carb. g
PANCAKES AND WAFFLES				
(See Condiments below for addition of butter & syrup.)				
Pancake (4" diam)				
Blueberry (1)	64	1	0	12
Buckwheat (1)	85	1	0	16
Plain (1)	74	1	0	14
Waffle (10" round)	665	38	11	67
CEREALS				
Cooked cereal, most brands (1 c)	145	2	0	25
Dry cereal, most types (1 single serving box or about 1 c)	110	2	0	22
Granola (1 c)	372	5	1	78
SIDE DISHES				
Bacon (2 sl)	73	6	2	0
Canadian bacon (1 oz)	58	3	1	0
Grits, plain (1 c)	181	4	1	32
Ham slice (3 oz)	170	10	3	0
Hash-brown potatoes (1 c)	321	17	4	41
Sausage links (2)	121	11	4	0
Sausage patties (2)	252	23	9	0
CONDIMENTS				
Butter (1 pat or 1 tsp)	34	4	2	0
Honey (1 Tbsp)	64	0	0	17
Jelly (1 Tbsp)	52	0	0	13
Margarine (1 pat or 1 tsp)	23	2	0	0
Syrup, maple & fruit flavors (1 Tbsp)	55	0	0	15

LUNCH AND DINNER

Choosing a restaurant at which many of the dishes are cooked to order instead of being prepared ahead of time gives you more control over how food is prepared. The following tips on lower-fat eating in a table-service (sit-down) restaurant apply to many types of eating establishments, ranging from fine dining to neighborhood cafés.

> **TIPS ON ORDERING LOWER-FAT FOOD AT LUNCH AND DINNER**
>
> - Read the menu carefully and ask how the food is prepared, paying special attention to terms indicating high fat (see page 7) or high sodium (see page 8).
> - Be assertive! Tell your server how you want your food prepared.
> - To get only the food you want, order à la carte instead of ordering a set meal with its accompaniments.
> - Don't hesitate to ask for substitutions, such as a baked potato, vegetables, carrot sticks, or a tossed salad instead of French fries; many restaurants do not charge for substitutions if the requested item is on the menu.
> - Order two low-fat appetizers in place of an entrée.
> - Split an entrée with a dining companion; you may each wish to order a separate salad and vegetables.
> - If a restaurant serves large portions, ask for a carryout container so that you can take home the uneaten part of your meal.
> - "Diet plates" are not always low in saturated fat and calories; ask what is included and how the food is prepared.
> - Cafeterias, delicatessens, and buffets allow you to see food before selecting or ordering it. Looking at all the foods being offered before you start down the cafeteria line or place your order in a deli will help you select those that are lower in fat and saturated fat.
>
> *(continued)*

TIPS ON ORDERING LOWER-FAT FOOD AT LUNCH AND DINNER *(continued)*

- At a buffet, walk around the table, decide which four or five foods are the lowest in fat, and select those instead of taking some of everything that is offered; do not go back for second helpings.
- Eat slowly to control the amount of food you consume.
- Remember, you do not have to clean your plate.

APPETIZERS AND SOUPS

> ### TIPS ON SELECTING
> ### LOWER-FAT APPETIZERS AND SOUPS
>
> - Order appetizers that are not fried.
> - Select soups with clear broth, such as chicken noodle or vegetable, instead of cream soup.

> ### TIP ON LOWERING SODIUM
>
> - Order fruit or salad instead of soup as an appetizer.

The following table gives you an idea of the calories, fat, saturated fat, and carbohydrate content of selected lunch and dinner foods. These values are only estimates, and the content of an actual dish may vary, depending on how the chef prepares it. Usually foods lower in fat are also lower in calories and saturated fat.

	Calories	Sat. Fat g	Fat g	Carb. g
APPETIZERS				
Buffalo chicken wings (10)	852	61	20	32
w/blue cheese dip (¼ c)	1109	87	22	38
Chile con queso (½ c)	200	16	9	6
w/tortilla chips (12)	309	21	10	20
Crab cakes, 2 (3½" diam)	520	33	8	26
Egg roll (4" long)	373	17	4	41
Fried calamari (3 oz)	300	15	3	22
Fried cheese, 2 pieces (4" x 1" x ¾")	409	31	17	12
Fried mushrooms (6)	199	10	2	22
Nachos w/beans & cheese (6)	198	9	4	20
Oysters, fried (6)	238	13	3	19
Potato wedges (6)	101	5	1	14
Topped w/cheese, sour cream & bacon	321	24	12	15
Prosciutto (½ oz) & honeydew melon (1 sl)	120	4	1	15
Shrimp cocktail (6 lg shrimp)	107	1	0	19

	Calories	Fat g	Sat. Fat g	Carb. g
Shrimp, bacon-wrapped (6)	262	20	7	0
Shrimp, fried (6)	125	6	1	8
Smoked salmon (1 oz)	33	1	0	0
Spinach dip (½ c)	231	20	6	12
w/tortilla chips (12)	340	25	7	26

SOUPS

	Calories	Fat g	Sat. Fat g	Carb. g
Baked potato soup (1 c)	317	18	10	24
Beef w/vegetables (1 c)	71	2	1	9
Black bean (1 c)	186	5	2	25
Broccoli cheese (1 c)	179	11	5	13
Chicken (1 c)	77	2	1	12
Chicken noodle (1 c)	76	3	1	9
Cream of mushroom (1 c)	110	7	2	9
Gazpacho (1 c)	87	5	1	12
Gumbo w/seafood & rice (1 c)	313	17	5	20
Manhattan clam chowder, tomato base (1 c)	73	2	1	12
Minestrone (1 c)	92	2	1	15
New England clam chowder, cream base (1 c)	244	15	3	21
Potato (1 c)	212	14	4	16
Split pea w/bacon (1 c)	181	4	1	26
Tomato bisque (1 c)	202	7	4	30
Tortilla soup (1 c)	145	10	5	6
Vegetarian vegetable (1 c)	74	0	0	17

SALADS AND SALAD BARS

Many people assume that all foods from a salad bar are low in calories and fat; however, some salad bar selections are high in both. A salad bar gives you the advantage of selecting specific low-fat foods and controlling the amount of each food.

TIPS ON SELECTING LOWER-FAT SALADS

- Select more fresh vegetables and fruits and fewer prepared salads, such as pasta, chicken, tuna, and potato salads.
- Add a serving of marinated vegetables on top of your salad instead of regular dressing; the marinade will drip throughout and flavor the salad greens.
- Request reduced calorie salad dressing.
- Order salad dressing on the side. To add it to your salad, dip your fork into the dressing, then into the salad, and then into your mouth.

TIPS ON LOWERING SODIUM

- Eat plain, raw vegetables instead of pickled vegetables.
- Select fresh vegetables and fruit instead of prepared salads, such as chicken, tuna, potato, and pasta salads, which are higher in sodium.
- Use lemon juice, vinegar, or oil and vinegar (from separate bottles) instead of prepared dressings on salad.

	Calories	Fat g	Sat. Fat g	Carb. g
SALAD BAR				
Bean sprouts (½ c)	9	0	0	2
Beets, sliced (½ c)	29	0	0	7
Broccoli, raw (½ c pieces)	10	0	0	2
Carrots, raw (½ c sl)	13	0	0	3
Cauliflower, raw (1 c pieces)	13	0	0	3

	Calories	Fat g	Sat. Fat g	Carb. g
Cucumber, raw slices (¼ c)	3	0	0	1
Garbanzo beans/chickpeas (¼ c)	67	1	0	11
Green beans, marinated (¼ c)	17	1	0	2
Kidney beans (¼ c)	56	0	0	10
Mushrooms, marinated (¼ c)	14	1	0	1
Mushrooms, raw (¼ sl)	4	0	0	1
Spinach, raw (1 c)	7	0	0	1
Tomato, cherry (4)	14	0	0	3
Tossed salad w/tomatoes & carrots	28	0	0	6

PREPARED SALADS

	Calories	Fat g	Sat. Fat g	Carb. g
Caesar salad w/dressing (3 c)	467	38	8	17
w/chicken (1 breast)	657	45	10	17
Carrot & raisin salad w/mayo dressing (½ c)	158	10	1	18
Chef's salad (3 c) w/turkey (1½ oz), ham (1½ oz), cheese (1½ oz), egg (1) & no dressing	387	23	11	12
Chicken salad w/egg & mayo dressing (½ c)	169	10	2	5
Cole slaw w/mayo dressing (½ c)	157	13	2	10
Fruit salad fresh (½ c)	92	1	0	23
Fruit salad w/whipped topping & marshmallows (½ c)	58	1	1	13
Gelatin w/cottage cheese & fruit (½ c)	107	2	1	15
Gelatin w/fruit (½ c)	68	0	0	17
Grilled chicken salad (1 breast) w/o croutons, no dressing	195	6	2	6
Pasta salad, w/o meat or cheese, w/Italian dressing (½ c)	67	3	0	10
Pea salad w/cheese & mayo dressing (½ c)	215	16	6	10
Potato salad w/egg & mayo dressing (½ c)	168	11	2	14
Shrimp salad w/egg & mayo dressing (½ c)	191	14	2	4

	Calories	Fat g	Sat. Fat g	Carb. g
Tabouli (½ c)	79	6	1	6
Three-bean salad w/oil dressing (½ c)	138	11	2	8
Tuna salad w/egg & mayo dressing (½ c)	191	13	2	6
Waldorf salad (½ c)	137	11	2	9

SALAD DRESSING

	Calories	Fat g	Sat. Fat g	Carb. g
Blue cheese or Roquefort (¼ c)	257	26	2	6
Caesar (¼ c)	208	22	4	2
French (¼ c)	226	20	3	14
Honey mustard (¼ c)	200	20	3	6
Italian (¼ c)	246	25	2	6
Fat-free (¼ c)	21	0	0	6
Reduced-calorie (¼ c)	84	8	1	4
Olive oil (1 Tbsp)	119	14	2	0
Thousand Island (¼ c)	206	21	4	4
Vinegar & oil (¼ c)	246	25	2	6

EXTRAS

	Calories	Fat g	Sat. Fat g	Carb. g
American cheese, grated (¼ c)	114	9	6	0
Bacon bits (1 Tbsp)				
Imitation	22	0	0	1
Real	27	2	1	0
Black olive slices (¼ c)	42	4	1	2
Cottage cheese, regular or creamed (½ c)	109	5	3	3
Croutons (½ c)	93	4	1	13
Parmesan cheese (1 Tbsp)	28	2	1	0
Pickle, dill (6 sl)	8	0	0	2
Sunflower seeds (1 Tbsp)	51	4	1	2

ENTRÉES

Most fish and poultry without skin (cooked without added fat) are lower in fat than red meat. Most fish is naturally low in fat; any fat found in fish is rich in polyunsaturated fat, which does not cause an increase in blood cholesterol levels. Many chefs increase the amount of fat in meat, poultry, and fish dishes during preparation by sautéing, pan-frying, breading and deep-frying, adding sauce, and basting before and during broiling and grilling. Meat, poultry, and fish that is "broiled" in a restaurant is often cooked with a generous amount of butter or margarine to prevent it from drying out. Weights of meat, poultry, and fish given on restaurant menus are for the raw meat; allow for 25% weight loss during cooking. (In the following table, weights are given for raw meat.)

> ## TIPS ON ORDERING
> ## LOWER-FAT ENTRÉES
>
> - Select roasted, grilled, or baked meats instead of fried meat or casseroles, which are usually high in fat because of the ground meat, butter, sour cream, oil, and/or cheese in them.
> - Select lean red meats, such as sirloin or tenderloin of beef, filet mignon (without bacon), loin pork chops, ham steak, or leg of lamb with the fat cut off, rather than higher-fat cuts, such as prime rib, prime steaks, T-bone steaks, rib-eye steaks, or ribs.
> - Ask that meat fat and poultry skin be removed before cooking.
> - Ask that a very small amount of oil or no oil be used in sautéing or stir-frying foods; request that meat, poultry, and fish be broiled or grilled without added fat.
> - Requesting that fish be "broiled dry" may not result in a tasty entrée—instead, ask to have your fish "baked with a splash of wine," "poached," or "shallow poached" (partially cooked on top of stove and finished in the oven).
> - Select entrées without rich sauce or cheese, or ask that sauce or gravy for meat, fish, or poultry be served in a side dish so that you can control the amount eaten.

TIPS ON LOWERING SODIUM

- Choose cooked-to-order dishes and ask that they be prepared without salt, MSG (monosodium glutamate), or soy sauce. Sodium in food prepared ahead of time, including soups, sauces, gravies, and casseroles, cannot be reduced.
- Use lemon instead of cocktail or tartar sauce with fish.

	Calories	Fat g	Sat. Fat g	Carb. g
FISH AND SHELLFISH				
Weight is for fish before cooking (raw).				
Catfish, fried (8 oz)	835	48	10	45
Catfish, grilled (8 oz)	374	20	4	0
Flounder, grilled (8 oz)	226	6	2	0
Salmon, grilled (8 oz)	366	18	5	0
Salmon, poached, no fat or sauce (8 oz)	323	13	4	0
Shrimp, fried (8 large)	166	8	2	11
Snapper, grilled (8 oz)	245	7	2	0
CHICKEN				
Chicken, BBQ, w/skin (half chicken)	555	23	6	29
Chicken breast, fried w/skin	479	26	6	25
Chicken breast, grilled w/o skin	190	7	2	0
w/skin	228	11	3	0
Chicken potpie (8 oz)	336	18	6	25
Chicken thigh & drumstick, fried w/skin	714	44	11	33
BEEF				
Weight is for beef before cooking (raw) except as noted.				
Beef Stroganoff w/noodles (1 c)	369	18	7	33
Chicken fried steak (8 oz)	865	54	16	39
w/cream gravy (½ c)	1056	69	21	47
Chili, no beans (1 c)	217	12	5	14
Chopped beefsteak (8 oz)	472	35	14	0

Entrées

	Calories	Fat g	Sat. Fat g	Carb. g
Filet mignon (no bacon wrap) or tenderloin, fat trimmed off (8 oz)	388	20	7	0
Fat & bacon wrap eaten	593	44	16	0
Meat loaf (8 oz cooked)	503	28	11	24
Pot roast of beef, fat trimmed off (8 oz cooked)	668	46	16	0
Fat eaten	762	59	24	0
Rib eye steak, fat eaten (8 oz)	524	38	14	0
Ribs, beef, fat eaten (8 oz)	562	42	17	3
Sirloin steak, fat trimmed off (8 oz)	288	10	3	0
Fat eaten	470	30	11	0
Stuffed green peppers (2)	576	26	11	48
T-bone steak, fat trimmed off (8 oz)	388	20	7	0
Fat eaten	524	38	14	0
Veal steak, fat trimmed off (8 oz)	244	11	4	0

PORK

Weight is for pork before cooking (raw).

	Calories	Fat g	Sat. Fat g	Carb. g
Pork chops, butterfly (8 oz)	490	31	11	0
Pork tenderloin, no visible fat eaten (8 oz cooked)	372	11	4	0
Ribs, pork, country style, fat eaten (8 oz)	593	47	17	0

SANDWICHES

TIPS ON ORDERING A LOWER-FAT SANDWICH

- Choose a prepared-to-order sandwich, which allows you more control over ingredients, rather than one prepared ahead of time. Request toppings, such as lettuce, tomato, pickles, and onion, instead of bacon and cheese; bread, a bun, or a roll instead of a croissant; and mustard or catsup instead of mayonnaise.
- Select lean roast beef, lean ham, sliced turkey or chicken, or grilled chicken, which are lower in fat than hamburgers or mixed-filling sandwiches (tuna, chicken, ham, or egg salad).
- When ordering a hamburger, choose one with a small meat patty and add lettuce, tomato, pickle, and onion instead of selecting one with a large patty or double meat.
- When ordering a submarine or po-boy sandwich, choose turkey, lean ham, or lean roast beef instead of cold cuts, and omit the cheese and the oil-and-vinegar dressing that is often sprinkled on top.
- Split a large sandwich with a friend by ordering extra bread and sharing the meat.
- Remove the top piece of bread from a sandwich and eat it "open-face" to decrease calories.
- Order a deli "lite" sandwich, which usually contains less meat than a regular sandwich.

TIPS ON LOWERING SODIUM

- Select grilled chicken instead of cold cuts and cheese, which are higher in sodium.
- If "fresh" cooked turkey is available, choose it instead of "deli-type" sliced turkey and roast beef, which are processed with sodium.
- If a sandwich comes with chips, ask that carrot sticks, fruit, or a salad be substituted.
- Request sweet pickles, which are much lower in sodium than dill or sour pickles.

Sandwich shops and delis vary in the amount of meat or mixed filling such as pimento cheese and (chicken, tuna, egg, and ham salads) they use in a sandwich. A sliced meat sandwich may contain 2 to 7 oz meat, or even more.

	Calories	Fat g	Sat. Fat g	Carb. g
COLD SANDWICHES				
Bologna (1 oz) & cheese (1 oz) w/stick margarine on bread	364	23	9	26
Corned beef (2 oz) sandwich	278	10	4	26
Ham (1 oz) & cheese (2 oz) w/stick margarine on bread	376	20	8	25
Roast beef (3 oz) & Swiss cheese (1 oz) sandwich	423	20	9	25
Submarine or hoagie w/cold cuts & condiments	335	10	3	42
Turkey (3 oz) w/mayo on bread	344	14	3	25
MIXED-FILLING SANDWICHES (4 oz filling, 2 sl bread)				
Chicken salad	407	20	4	35
Egg salad	441	28	5	32
Ham salad	449	28	5	32
Pimento cheese	422	24	14	40
Tuna salad	372	18	3	34
HOT SANDWICHES				
Bacon, lettuce & tomato w/mayo on bread	286	16	4	28
BBQ beef (1½ oz) on a bun	358	13	5	46
Chicken fillet, breaded (2 oz) on a bun w/lettuce, tomato & mayo	484	29	6	27
Club w/bacon (2 sl), turkey (2 oz), tomato & mayo on bread (3 sl)	480	23	5	40
Denver or Western w/egg, ham, onion & green pepper on bread (2 sl)	312	16	4	28
Fish, fried (1½ oz) w/tartar sauce on a bun	417	19	4	43
Grilled cheese (1 oz cheese)	304	18	7	25
Gyro w/beef & lamb (1 oz) & condiments in pita bread	257	15	3	19

	Calories	Fat g	Sat. Fat g	Carb. g
Hot dog (1½ oz wiener) on a bun w/chili & cheese	440	26	12	32
Monte Cristo w/ham (1 oz), cheese (1 oz) & bread (2 sl), egg-dipped & fried	423	24	12	29
Reuben w/corned beef (2 oz), sauerkraut, cheese (1 oz) & dressing on rye bread (2 sl), grilled	516	33	11	30
Roast beef (3 oz) w/gravy on bread (2 sl)	391	17	6	29

HAMBURGERS (see Chapter 4)

	Calories	Fat g	Sat. Fat g	Carb. g
Cheeseburger, single meat patty w/mayo	388	26	8	22
w/bacon (3 sl)	497	35	12	22
Hamburger, single meat patty w/catsup	252	11	4	26

SPREADS

	Calories	Fat g	Sat. Fat g	Carb. g
Catsup (1 Tbsp)	16	0	0	4
Mayonnaise (1 Tbsp)	74	7	1	2
Mustard (1 Tbsp)	10	0	0	1

SANDWICH EXTRAS

	Calories	Fat g	Sat. Fat g	Carb. g
Cheddar cheese (1 oz)	114	9	6	0
Corn chips (1 oz bag)	155	10	1	14
Dill pickle spear (1)	5	0	0	1
French fries (lg order)	515	26	6	67
Lettuce leaf (1)	1	0	0	0
Oil & vinegar dressing drizzled over sandwich (1 Tbsp)	62	6	1	1
Onion rings (12 lg)	347	23	7	33
Onion slice (2)	7	0	0	2
Pickle, sweet (1 med)	29	0	0	8
Potato chips (1 oz bag)	156	10	2	16
Swiss cheese (1 oz)	107	8	5	1
Tomato slices (2)	6	0	0	1

	Calories	Fat g	Sat. Fat g	Carb. g
BREADS AND ROLLS				
Bread				
Rye (2 sl)	135	2	0	25
White (2 sl)	134	2	0	25
Whole wheat (2 sl)	139	2	0	26
Croissant (4½")	259	15	9	27
Submarine or hoagie roll (8" long)	258	3	1	49

PIZZA

TIPS ON ORDERING LOWER-FAT PIZZA

- Eat a large salad before eating pizza to take the edge off your appetite.
- Order a vegetarian rather than a meat pizza.
- Request less cheese or no cheese on your pizza.
- If you want meat, request it on half of the pizza. Canadian bacon is usually the leanest type of meat available.
- Thin-crust pizza has less fat in the crust than rising pizza crust. Deep-dish pizza may have extra cheese and meat toppings, making it even higher in fat and saturated fat than rising crust pizza.
- Avoid "stuffed" or "filled" pizzas and side orders such as cheese bread, cinnamon bread sticks, and buffalo wings.

TIPS ON LOWERING SODIUM

- Request that little or no cheese be used on the pizza.
- Select vegetable toppings (except olives), which are lower in sodium than meat toppings.
- Request that anchovies not be added to your pizza.

VEGETABLES

TIPS ON ORDERING LOWER-FAT VEGETABLES

- Top a baked potato with chives or green onions, catsup, lemon juice, jalapeño peppers, mustard, salsa, or a small amount of margarine or low-fat ranch or French dressing. Potatoes that are French-fried, creamed, hash-browned, escalloped, au gratin, mashed, stuffed, or twice baked are high in fat and saturated fat.
- Select foods without rich sauce or cheese.

TIPS ON LOWERING SODIUM

- Order vegetables without sauce or cheese.
- Select a baked potato and add green onion, lemon juice, chives, or a small amount of margarine.

	Calories	Fat g	Sat. Fat g	Carb. g
VEGETABLES				
Asparagus seasoned w/ margarine (¾ c)	63	3	1	7
Baked beans (¾ c)				
w/bacon	377	12	4	56
w/franks	271	10	4	35
Boston baked beans (¾ c)	679	26	3	99
Broccoli seasoned w/ margarine (4 florets)	19	1	0	2
Broccoli w/cheese sauce (¾ c)	186	12	6	10
Brussels sprouts, seasoned w/ margarine (¾ c)	75	3	1	10
Cabbage seasoned w/bacon (¾ c)	50	3	1	5
Carrots, glazed, seasoned w/ margarine (¾ c)	104	4	1	16
Cauliflower seasoned w/ margarine (¾ c)	43	3	1	4

	Calories	Fat g	Sat. Fat g	Carb. g
Cauliflower w/cheese sauce (¾ c)	178	13	7	8
Corn on the cob w/margarine (7" long)	152	6	1	25
Corn, whole kernel, seasoned w/margarine (¾ c)	124	3	1	24
French fries (10)	140	8	2	17
Green beans seasoned w/ margarine (¾ c)	54	3	1	7
Green bean casserole w/cheese & cream of mushroom soup (¾ c)	272	19	9	15
Mixed vegetables, broccoli, cauliflower & carrots seasoned w/margarine (¾ c)	44	3	1	4
Mushrooms sautéed in butter (¾ c)	57	3	2	6
Okra, cornmeal dipped & fried (¾ c)	128	6	1	15
Okra, steamed, seasoned w/ margarine (¾ c)	59	3	1	7
Peas, green, seasoned w/ margarine (¾ c)	119	3	1	17
Pinto beans w/bacon (¾ c)	198	3	1	33
Potato, baked (1 lg)	150	0	0	35
Bacon, crumbled (2 Tbsp)	54	3	1	0
Butter (3 pats)	102	12	7	0
Cheese, grated (¼ c)	114	9	6	0
Sour cream (2 Tbsp)	56	6	3	1
Potato w/all trimmings listed above	476	30	17	36
Potatoes, au gratin, w/cheese sauce (¾ c)	314	19	9	25
Potatoes, mashed, seasoned w/margarine (¾ c)	194	9	2	27
Potatoes, roasted, w/margarine (¾ c pieces)	104	3	1	18
Potatoes, sweet, candied, seasoned w/margarine (¾ c)	263	6	1	51

	Calories	Fat g	Sat. Fat g	Carb. g
Spinach, seasoned w/margarine (¾ c)	63	3	1	7
Spinach w/butter sauce (¾ c)	65	3	2	8
Spinach, creamed (¾ c)	111	6	2	10
Squash casserole w/cheese, milk & margarine (¾ c)	431	31	11	26
Turnip greens seasoned w/ bacon (¾ c)	50	3	1	5
Zucchini seasoned w/ margarine (¾ c)	47	3	1	5

BREADS AND CRACKERS

> **TIPS ON ORDERING LOWER-FAT BREADS**
>
> - Select French bread, hard rolls, hard breadsticks, saltine crackers, or sliced bread, which are lower in fat than cornbread, muffins, and dinner rolls (brushed with margarine or butter).
> - Eat bread, rolls, and crackers without butter or margarine.

> **TIP ON LOWERING SODIUM**
>
> - Yeast breads, such as sliced bread and hard rolls, are lower in sodium than breads containing baking powder, such as biscuits and cornbread.

	Calories	Fat g	Sat. Fat g	Carb. g
BREADS				
Cornbread (3" x 3" x 1")	190	6	2	29
French hard roll (1 med)	147	2	0	26
Garlic bread, buttered (1 lg sl)	366	15	3	49
Hot roll (1 med)	108	3	1	18
White bread (1 sl)	80	1	0	15

(See also Baked Goods, page 14.)

CRACKERS				
Breadstick, cracker type (6½" long)	159	5	1	25
Melba toast (2 rectangles)	39	0	0	8
Saltines (3)	40	1	0	6
SPREADS				
Butter (1 pat)	34	4	2	0
Margarine (1 pat)	34	4	1	0

DESSERTS

> **TIPS ON ORDERING LOWER-FAT DESSERTS**
>
> - Skip dessert, split a serving with your dinner companion, or select fruit, angel food cake, sherbet, frozen yogurt, or gelatin (without sour cream, cream cheese, or whipped topping) instead of pie, cake, cookies, mousse, cheesecake, or ice cream. Most of the fat in fruit pie and cobbler is in the crust—reduce the fat by eating the filling and only a small amount of the crust. Most whipped toppings are high in fat and saturated fat, even those labeled "nondairy."
> - Eat cake without frosting.

> **TIP ON LOWERING SODIUM**
>
> - Select fruit, gelatin, frozen yogurt, or sherbet instead of a baked dessert.

	Calories	Fat g	Sat. Fat g	Carb. g
DESSERTS				
Cakes				
Angel food, plain (1/12 of cake)	141	0	0	32
w/frosting	393	9	8	76
Applesauce w/cream cheese frosting (1/8 of 9" 2-layer cake)	699	26	10	110
Carrot w/cream cheese frosting (1/8 of 9" 2-layer cake)	730	28	10	115
Cheesecake (1/8 of 9" diam x 1½" ht)	629	45	23	49
Chocolate w/chocolate butter cream frosting (1/8 of 9" 2-layer cake)	731	37	19	102
Fudge w/cream cheese frosting (1/8 of 9" 2-layer cake)	708	27	10	113

	Calories	Fat g	Sat. Fat g	Carb. g
Pineapple upside-down (3" x 3" x 2" ht)	372	17	3	52
Pound w/frosting (5" x 3" x 1")	646	33	18	83
Strawberry shortcake (2½" diam) w/whipped topping	194	9	3	27
Frozen yogurt, low-fat (¾ c)	147	2	1	28
Gelatin, plain (¾ c)	95	0	0	23
w/fruit & cream cheese whipped topping	57	2	1	10
Ice cream, chocolate (¾ c)	268	18	11	25
Sundae w/fudge sauce, nuts & whipped cream	463	27	13	52
Petit four (1"x1"x1")	39	2	1	5
Pies (⅛ of 9" pie)				
Apple, double-crust	369	15	4	56
Banana cream	377	19	7	45
Cherry, double-crust	330	13	3	52
Chocolate cream w/whipped topping	257	15	7	28
Coconut cream	330	17	7	38
Lemon meringue	403	15	5	64
Strawberry w/glaze, w/o whipped topping	216	7	2	39
w/whipped topping	293	13	6	43
Sherbet (¾ c)	153	2	1	34
Strawberries, halves (1 c)	46	1	0	11

BEVERAGES

In restaurants across the US, a wide variety of beverages are served with meals and between meals. A popular trend as been flavored coffees, served in specialty coffee shops, as well as restaurants, and fast food places.

A recent trend is bubble tea, also known as pearl tea, tapioca tea, boba, and milk tea, which contains brewed black or green tea, tapioca pearls, milk and honey or sugar, and may include blended fruit juice and other flavorings. Calories and fat vary depending on the size of cup, the type of milk (whole, low-fat, or fat-free), the amount of juice (if any), and the amount of pearl tapioca (primarily carbohydrate) used.

> **TIPS ON ORDERING BEVERAGES**
>
> - Ask for water if it is not provided.
> - Choose milk that is skim or fat free, 1/2%, or 1% low-fat.
> - Sparkling water, seltzer, and calorie-free soft drinks are refreshing while providing no calories.
> - Drink calorie-free beverages before and during the meal to reduce your hunger and help you feel satisfied.
> - For low-calorie lemonade, squeeze lemon slices into a glass of ice water and add sugar substitute.

Alcoholic Beverages

Alcoholic beverages are high in calories, can increase your appetite, and tend to decrease your willpower. If you drink alcoholic beverages, do so in moderation, which is no more than 2 drinks for men and 1 drink for women and older people per day. Children, adolescents, and pregnant women should not drink alcohol.

ONE DRINK IS DEFINED AS:

- 5 fl oz of wine
- 12 fl oz of beer (regular or lite)
- 1½ oz (80 proof) of whiskey, rum, gin, scotch, or vodka

Most alcoholic drinks do not contain fat; however, fat is added to some mixed drinks in the form of cream, eggs, whole milk, or cream of coconut, and a few bottled alcoholic drinks contain cream.

	Calories	Fat g	Sat. Fat g	Carb. g
CARBONATED DRINKS (12 fl oz)				
Club soda	0	0	0	0
Cola	153	0	0	39
Diet cola	4	0	0	0
Ginger ale	146	0	0	38
Orange soda	147	0	0	38
COFFEE				
Black (8 fl oz)	5	0	0	1
w/half & half (1 Tbsp)	20	2	1	1
w/sugar (1 pkt)	23	0	0	6
Café au lait (16 fl oz)				
w/skim milk	126	0	0	26
w/whole milk	161	4	3	26
Café latte (16 fl oz)				
w/skim milk	212	1	0	40
w/whole milk	306	12	7	39
Cappuccino (16 fl oz)				
w/skim milk	193	1	0	35
w/whole milk	281	11	7	35
FRUIT DRINKS (8 fl oz)				
Cranberry juice cocktail	144	0	0	36
Fruit punch	116	1	0	26
MILK AND MILK-BASED DRINKS				
Chocolate milkshake (12 fl oz)	309	8	5	52
Cocoa (1 pkg mix) prep w/water	138	1	0	32
Eggnog w/o alcohol (8 fl oz)	342	19	11	34
Milk (8 fl oz)				
½% fat	92	1	1	12
1% fat	102	3	2	12
2% fat	121	5	3	12
Chocolate	208	8	5	26
Skim	86	0	0	12
Whole	150	8	5	11

	Calories	Fat g	Sat. Fat g	Carb. g
TEA (8 fl oz)				
Tea, unsweetened	2	0	0	1
w/sugar (2 pkt)	46	0	0	12
ALCOHOLIC BEVERAGES				
Beer (12 fl oz)	146	0	0	13
"Near" beer, no alcohol	146	0	0	37
Lite	99	0	0	5
Black Russian (2¼ fl oz)	160	0	0	12
Bloody Mary (8 fl oz)	160	0	0	8
Bourbon and soda (4 fl oz)	96	0	0	0
Brandy Alexander (4 fl oz)	252	5	3	24
Champagne (6 fl oz)	120	0	0	1
Daiquiri, frozen (4 fl oz)	62	0	0	7
Not frozen (4 fl oz)	246	0	0	7
Gin (1½ fl oz)	96	0	0	0
Gin and tonic (4 fl oz)	89	0	0	10
Grasshopper (4 fl oz)	274	5	3	37
Hot buttered rum (4 fl oz)	146	6	3	2
Irish coffee (8 fl oz)	155	4	3	8
Long Island iced tea (4 fl oz)	110	0	0	9
Manhattan (4 fl oz)	215	0	0	3
Margarita, not frozen (8 fl oz)	492	0	0	14
Martini (4 fl oz)	222	0	0	0
Mimosa (8 fl oz)	142	0	0	9
Piña colada (12 fl oz)	599	23	20	79
Rum (1½ fl oz)	96	0	0	0
Rum and cola (4 fl oz)	91	0	0	9
Rum punch (4 fl oz)	128	0	0	9
Scotch and soda (4 fl oz)	96	0	0	0
Screwdriver (8 fl oz)	207	0	0	18
Vodka (1½ fl oz)	96	0	0	0
Vodka Collins (4 fl oz)	74	0	0	3
Vodka tonic (12 fl oz)	231	0		
Whiskey (1½ fl oz)	96	0	0	0
Wine				
Dessert or sweet (2 fl oz)	90	0	0	7
Red (6 fl oz)	127	0	0	3
White (6 fl oz)	120	0	0	1

SNACKS

Eating away from home can include snacks as well as meals. For some people, food eaten as snacks makes up a significant amount of the calories, fat, and saturated fat consumed each day. Snacking ranges from eating ice cream at a specialty shop, popcorn at a movie theater, and peanuts at a ball game to buying pretzels and a soft drink or picking up a candy bar for quick energy. You can also find foods consumed as snacks in Chapter 4 on fast food.

	Calories	Fat g	Sat. Fat g	Carb. g
SNACKS				
Brownie w/nuts & frosting (3" x 3" x 1")	545	34	13	61
Cappuccino, bottled (1 lg)	511	8	5	99
Caramels (3 = 1 oz)	116	2	2	23
Chips (1 oz)				
Corn chips (30)	145	10	1	13
Pork skins (30)	164	9	3	0
Potato chips (20)	154	10	2	16
Tortilla chips (16)	146	7	1	18
Cookies (4" diam x ½")				
Chocolate chip	388	17	6	53
Oatmeal	293	13	5	40
Peanut butter	361	20	5	43
Sugar	252	12	3	32
Frozen fruit & juice bar (1)	53	0	0	14
Granola bars (1 = 1 oz)				
Plain	94	4	2	14
Cereal bar	140	3	0	27
Chocolate-coated	139	7	4	17
Ice cream pie, chocolate w/pie crust (⅛ of 9")	366	23	11	37
Ice cream, rich (1 c)	355	19	12	42
In waffle cone	372	20	12	45
In sugar cone	476	21	12	65
Jelly beans (10 = 1 oz)	110	0	0	28
Jerky, beef (8½" x 1" x ⅛") (2 strips = 1½ oz)	162	10	4	4

	Calories	Fat g	Sat. Fat g	Carb. g
Milk chocolate candy, plain (1½ oz = 1 bar)	225	13	8	26
Milkshake, chocolate (16 fl oz)	412	11	7	69
Peanuts, dry-roasted (¼ c)	212	18	3	7
Popcorn (4 cups popped)				
Not "buttered"	221	12	2	25
w/"butter"	424	35	7	25
Pretzels, rings (25 sm = 1 oz)	114	1	0	24
Pudding, ready-to-eat (4 oz)	150	5	1	26
Rice cakes (3 w/4" diam)	104	1	0	22
Trail mix (1 oz)				
Nuts, seeds, dried fruit & candy	173	11	2	17
Yogurt, frozen, low-fat (1 c)	203	3	2	39

CHAPTER 3

ETHNIC CUISINES

Cuisines from a variety of cultures are very popular in the United States. The three most popular ethnic cuisines are Chinese, Italian, and Mexican.

Many ethnic cuisines are based on foods that are naturally low in fat and calories. However, the Americanized versions of these foreign dishes are often higher in fat, saturated fat, cholesterol, and calories than the original foods, since they contain increased amounts of meat, cheese, and fat and smaller portions of grains, legumes, and vegetables. It is estimated that almost one third of the entrées ordered in the United States have foreign origins.

This book includes information on 10 ethnic cuisines; from Cajun/Creole to Vietnamese. We analyzed recipes from cookbooks representing each cuisine; the resulting estimated calories and values for fat, saturated fat, and carbohydrate appear on the following pages. The tables contain dishes both low and high in saturated fat.

CAJUN AND CREOLE CUISINE

South Louisiana is renowned for its Cajun and Creole cuisine. The cooking styles are today very similar. Originally, Cajun fare was that of the French Acadians who settled the bayous and prairies of southwestern Louisiana, whereas Creole cooking developed as a blend of New Orleans French, African, and Caribbean traditions. American Indian, Spanish, and German traditions also made important contributions to the cuisines. Both styles use an array of spicy seasonings; feature rice in main and side dishes; and use roux as a base for many soups, stews, and gravies. Roux, which is flour and fat blended and cooked to a caramel brown, accounts for the high fat content of many dishes. Both Cajun and Creole cooks perpare gumbos, étouffées, jambalayas, and innumerable other dishes. Local ingredients such as crayfish (often boiled), crab, shrimp, oysters, and wild game are featured. Seafood is often fried. "Blackening" entrées, which is nontraditional, involves dipping the seafood or meat in butter or oil and seasoning and cooking it in a very hot skillet. Other popular dishes include sausages such an andouille, boudin blanc, and boudin rouge; rice and (brown) gravy or red beans and rice (a Caribbean borrowing); and sweets such as beignets (square fired doughnuts with powdered sugar), bread pudding, pralines, and Bananas Foster.

MENU TERMS THAT INDICATE HIGH FAT

- Dirty rice—Prepared with chicken gizzards, chicken livers, ground pork, and butter or other fat
- Gumbo, étouffée, sauces, and gravies made with roux (see description of roux above)
- Hush puppies—Deep-fried cornmeal batter

In restaurants, the easiest way to select foods low in saturated fat is to select foods low in total fat.

TIPS ON ORDERING
LOWER-FAT CAJUN AND CREOLE FOOD

- Order boiled and grilled seafood rather than fried seafood as an appetizer or an entrée. Ask that blackened entrées be prepared with as little fat as possible. Shrimp and crayfish are low in fat and saturated fat (if not fried).
- Request that sauces and gravies be served on the side or omitted.
- Creole and jambalaya dishes may be lower in fat than gumbo and étouffée, depending on how they are prepared.
- Request white rice, even if it is seasoned with oil, as a substitute for "dirty" rice.
- Select menu items that do not include sausage. Order red beans and rice without the sausage commonly served as an accompaniment.

TIPS ON LOWERING SODIUM

- Select boiled seafood as an appetizer.
- Order grilled seafood, chicken, or steak as an entrée and request that it be prepared without salt.
- The sodium in gumbo, étouffée, jambalaya, and creole dishes cannot be reduced, since these dishes are prepared ahead of time.

The following table gives you an idea of the calories, fat, saturated fat and carbohydrate content of selected foods from restaurants serving popularized versions of Cajun or Creole cuisine. These values are only estimates, and the content of a dish may vary, depending on how the chef prepares it.

	Calories	Fat g	Sat. Fat g	Carb. g
APPETIZERS				
Crayfish, boiled (12)	148	2	0	0

	Calories	Fat g	Sat. Fat g	Carb. g
Gumbo (2 c)				
Roux-based soup w/seafood & sausage served w/rice	625	34	9	40
Oysters on the half shell (12)	168	6	2	10
Shrimp, boiled (12 lg)	71	1	0	0
ENTRÉES				
Catfish, fried (8 oz)	835	48	10	45
Chicken creole (1 c)				
Spicy tomato sauce served				
w/rice (¾ c)	398	12	5	42
w/o rice	218	9	3	9
Red beans (2 c) seasoned				
w/bacon & sausage				
w/rice (1 c)	767	12	5	132
Shrimp creole (1 c)				
Spicy tomato sauce served				
w/rice (¾ c)	386	12	4	49
w/o rice	206	8	2	16
Shrimp étouffée (2 c)				
Roux-based sauce w/shrimp served w/rice (1 c)	788	17	4	99
Shrimp, fried (12 lg)	249	13	3	16
Shrimp jambalaya (3 c)				
Seasoned rice dish w/tomatoes & shrimp	874	26	14	82
ACCOMPANIMENTS				
Candied yams w/butter & brown sugar (1 c)	351	9	5	67
Dirty rice (1 c)	301	13	5	24
Rice seasoned w/butter (1 c)	239	4	3	45
Red beans seasoned w/bacon & sausage (2 c)	528	8	3	88
BREADS				
Cornbread (3" x 3" x 2")	484	16	5	73
Hushpuppies (6)				
Deep-fried cornmeal batter	397	18	5	50

	Calories	Fat g	Sat. Fat g	Carb. g
DESSERTS				
Bananas Foster	862	26	14	156
Bread pudding (1½ c) w/rum cream sauce (¼ c)	764	30	16	106
Chocolate mousse (1 c)	565	37	21	55
Pecan praline (2" diam) Candy made w/butter, sugar, cream & pecans	218	7	1	40

CHINESE CUISINE

Chinese food differs widely in flavor and fat content depending on the region of China where the dish originated. The dishes most Americans think of as Chinese come from the south (Canton) and are steamed or stir-fried. Szechwan or Hunan foods, from western and central China, may be higher in fat and tend to be spicy from the chili peppers in them. Although rice is the staple in the eastern and coastal regions (Shanghai), food from the north and northeast (Beijing/Peking) is likely to be served with dumplings. Items such as fried egg rolls and fried butterfly shrimp with sweet-and-sour sauce, which are high in fat, are basic fare in Chinese restaurants; however, they are not part of typical Chinese meals and were developed in the United States.

MENU TERMS THAT INDICATE HIGH FAT

- Crispy or fried—Food has been fried and is high in fat and trans fat
- Entrées with cashews or peanuts—Nuts often are deep-fried before being added to food
- Sweet-and-sour entrées—Pork, shrimp, or chicken deep-fried, then stir-fried with vegetables in more oil before the addition of sweet-and-sour sauce

---

In restaurants, the easiest way to have foods low in saturated fat is to select foods low in total fat.

TIPS ON ORDERING LOWER-FAT CHINESE FOOD

- Since most Chinese dishes are prepared as they are ordered, special requests can usually be managed; ask that less oil be used to stir-fry.
- Order fewer entrées than the number of people eating the meal; it is common practice for diners to share the generous portions served in many Chinese restaurants.

(continued)

TIPS ON ORDERING LOWER-FAT CHINESE FOOD *(continued)*

- Select steamed dumplings rather than egg rolls as an appetizer.
- Select dishes with lots of vegetables, such as chop suey with steamed rice.
- Steamed foods with a variety of sauces are better choices than fried items at dim sum lunches, which offer a variety of small appetizers.
- Eat the steamed rice served with most entrées instead of ordering fried rice.
- Order dishes with water chestnuts, which are fat-free, rather than with cashews or peanuts, which add fat.

TIPS ON LOWERING SODIUM

- Select steamed foods, such as dumplings or fish, and add sweet-and-sour sauce at the table.
- Ask that MSG (monosodium glutamate) not be used in food. MSG cannot be left out of commercially prepared sauces.
- Select entrées not prepared with oyster or bean sauce, which are high in sodium.
- Soy sauce, which is very high in sodium, is often used in stir-fried dishes; ask that it be omitted.
- Use sweet-and-sour sauce, plum sauce, or duck sauce instead of soy sauce at the table.

The following table gives you an idea of the calories, fat, saturated fat, and carbohydrate content of selected foods from Chinese cuisine. These values are only estimates, and the content of an actual dish may vary, depending on how the chef prepares it.

	Calories	Fat g	Sat. Fat g	Carb. g
APPETIZERS				
Egg rolls, 4" long (2)	398	20	5	41
Fried chicken wings (8)	681	49	16	25
Fried wonton (6)	397	19	4	48
Fried wonton w/cream cheese filling (8)	751	51	29	55
Ribs (4 small)	397	30	11	0
Steamed dumplings (6)	283	5	1	49
SOUPS				
Egg drop (1 c)	90	5	2	1
Hot-and-sour (1 c)	120	6	2	5
Wonton (1 c)	235	4	1	34
ENTRÉES				
Beef lo mein (2 c) w/vegetables & soft noodles	569	24	6	73
Beef w/vegetables (2 c)	610	34	10	29
w/white rice (1 c)	815	34	10	74
Chicken w/almonds (2 c)	625	29	6	29
w/white rice (1 c)	830	29	6	74
Chicken w/Chinese vegetables (2 c)	454	19	4	18
w/white rice (1 c)	659	19	4	63
Chop suey w/meat or seafood (2 c)	368	23	9	17
w/white rice (1 c)	573	23	9	62
Chow mein				
Chicken (2 c)	270	10	3	17
Shrimp (2 c)	192	5	1	17
Add crispy chow mein noodles (1 c)	237	14	2	26
General Tso chicken (2 c)	588	34	8	32
Moo goo gai pan Chicken stir-fried w/vegetables (2 c)	647	38	7	20
w/white rice (1 c)	852	38	7	65
Pork w/Chinese vegetables (2 c)	568	34	9	18
w/white rice (1 c)	773	34	9	63

	Calories	Fat g	Sat. Fat g	Carb. g
Shrimp w/Chinese vegetables (2 c)	347	14	2	18
w/white rice (1 c)	552	14	2	63
Shrimp w/snow peas (2 c)	347	14	2	18
w/white rice (1 c)	552	14	2	63
Sweet-and-sour meat dish Breaded & fried cubes of meat w/sweet & sour sauce				
w/chicken (2 c)	1143	52	13	85
w/shrimp (2 c)	678	31	8	59
Add white rice (1 c)	205	0	0	45
Vegetable lo mein (2 c)				
w/soft noodles	521	17	3	85

ACCOMPANIMENTS

	Calories	Fat g	Sat. Fat g	Carb. g
Fried rice (1 c)	223	8	2	31
White rice (1 c)	205	0	0	45

SAUCES

	Calories	Fat g	Sat. Fat g	Carb. g
Lobster sauce (¼ c)	101	7	2	3
Mustard sauce (¼ c)	97	9	1	5
Oyster sauce (¼ c)	33	0	0	7
Plum or Duck sauce (¼ c)	176	0	0	42
Sweet-and-sour sauce (¼ c)	81	2	0	16

DESSERTS

	Calories	Fat g	Sat. Fat g	Carb. g
Fortune cookie (1)	27	0	0	6

FRENCH CUISINE

Classic French cuisine is known for its rich dishes, in which sauce with butter is often a key ingredient. In 1972 a new movement started that rejected overly rich, complicated dishes not suitable for health-conscious individuals. Advocates of the "nouvelle cuisine" seek fresh ingredients, lighter dishes, and simpler cooking methods, including the use of lower-fat, lighter sauces based on meat juices, stocks, and spices. Rapid cooking without fat is often used in nouvelle cuisine. Foods offered by the "new cooks" include crisp vegetables, prepared to retain their natural flavors; thin-sliced meat with the fat trimmed off; airy mousses; vegetable purées; and light fruity sauces to accompany desserts. While nouvelle cuisine is no longer modish, its good influences remain in lighter fare and smaller portions. Most French restaurants offer a combination of nouvelle cuisine and traditional dishes.

MENU TERMS THAT INDICATE HIGH FAT

- Au gratin—Foods that are topped with cheese and, sometimes, butter
- Béarnaise—Classic sauce containing butter and egg yolk, which is served with grilled meat, fowl, and eggs
- Béchamel—Basic white sauce made of milk, flour, and butter
- Bordelaise—Sauce of red or white wine with bone marrow and chopped parsley
- Crème fraîche—Tangy heavy cream
- Hollandaise—Sauce made with butter, egg yolks, and lemon juice
- Mornay—Béchamel sauce with additional butter, grated Parmesan, Gruyère cheese, and, sometimes, egg yolk
- Pâté—Rich mixture or spread made of meat, poultry, game, fish, or vegetables; pâté de foie gras—a smooth, rich pâté made with goose liver

In restaurants, the easiest way to have foods low in saturated fat is to select foods low in total fat.

**TIPS ON ORDERING
LOWER-FAT FRENCH FOOD**

- Choosing simple dishes is the easiest way to keep your meal low in fat while enjoying French cuisine.
- If you order a dish with an added sauce, ask that it be served in a side dish so that you can control the amount you use. Usually wine sauces, such as bordelaise, are lower in fat than sauces containing butter, egg, and/or cheese. Avoid the common practice of soaking up rich sauces with bread.
- Select French bread rather than croissants.
- Often chefs add butter to sauces immediately before serving, significantly increasing the saturated fat in dishes such as moules marinière. Request that the chef not add extra butter or oil prior to serving.
- For dessert, choose sorbet, which is a water ice containing beaten egg white and flavored with fruit juice or purée or other flavoring.

TIP ON LOWERING SODIUM

- Choose cooked-to-order dishes, such as grilled fish and vegetables, and ask that salt be omitted during preparation.

The following table gives you an idea of the calories, fat, saturated fat, and carbohydrate content of selected foods from French cuisine. These values are only estimates, and the content of an actual dish may vary, depending on how the chef prepares it.

	Calories	Fat g	Sat. Fat g	Carb. g
HORS D'OEUVRE				
Escargots à la bourguignone				
Snails baked in shells w/garlic butter (6)	301	29	18	3
Melon au porto				
Cantaloupe wedge w/port	69	0	0	9
Moules marinière				
Mussels (6 lg) cooked w/shallots in wine and butter	368	30	18	9
Huitres fraîches				
Oysters on the half shell (6)	84	3	1	5
SOUPES ET POTAGES (SOUPS)				
Soupe à l'oignon gratinée (1½ c)				
Onion soup w/bread & Swiss cheese	389	16	8	44
Vichyssoise (1½ c)				
Chilled leek & potato cream soup	366	24	15	31
SALADES (SALADS)				
Salasa César (2 c)				
Caesar salad w/anchovies	310	25	5	12
Salade verte (2 c)				
Mixed green salad	17	0	0	3
w/vinaigrette dressing	79	6	1	4
POISSONS (FISH)				
Sole meunière (8 oz)				
Sautéed sole in butter sauce	464	34	20	1
Homard grillé au beurre				
Lobster (1 lb) w/herb butter	541	43	26	2
Saumon crôute raifort (8 oz)				
Salmon fillet smoked w/ horseradish crust	385	23	11	11
Thon grillé sur une pôelé de poivrons mélanges (8 oz)				
Tuna, grilled on bed of roasted peppers w/balsamic vinegar sauce	304	15	6	9

	Calories	Fat g	Sat. Fat g	Carb. g
VIANDES ET VOLAILLES (MEAT AND POULTRY)				
Boeuf bourguignon (2 c)				
Beef stew w/burgundy, onions, mushrooms & bacon	527	31	14	35
Coq au vin (2 c)				
Chicken stew w/wine, onion, mushrooms & bacon	410	16	4	28
Gigot d'agneau (8 oz)				
Leg of lamb	467	29	11	0
Magret de canard				
Breast of duck (2 split breasts) browned in goose fat	534	30	9	0
Paupiette de veau (8 oz)				
Rolled veal stuffed w/ground pork & sautéed in butter	545	33	15	12
Rôti de porc (8 oz)				
Roast loin of pork (fat trimmed off)	374	17	8	0
Steak au poivre (8 oz)				
Steak w/crushed peppercorns, pan-fried in butter	467	30	12	0
PAINS (BREADS)				
Butter (1 Tbsp)	102	12	7	0
Croissant (1 med)	259	15	9	27
French bread (1 med sl)	173	2	1	32
DESSERTS				
Mousse au chocolat (1 c)				
Chocolate mousse	565	37	21	55
Sorbet (½ c)	97	0	0	25
Tarte aux pommes (⅛ of 9" diam)				
Open-face apple pie	305	12	8	48

GREEK CUISINE

The cuisines of Greece and Middle Eastern countries share a number of common dishes. Many Greek and Middle Eastern dishes are high in fat because of the lavish use of oil, usually olive oil. Popular grain dishes include rice pilaf, couscous, and tabouli, which typically contain olive oil. Chickpeas are often puréed with fava beans to make falafel or mashed with sesame seed paste (tahini) to make hummus.

MENU TERMS THAT INDICATE HIGH FAT

- Baklava—Sweet dessert made of phyllo dough, honey, butter, and nuts
- Falafel—Deep-fried ball or patty of minced chickpeas and/or fava beans
- Feta—White, medium-fat goat's or sheep's milk cheese; when made outside Greece, it may be made from cow's milk or a combination of cow's and goat's milk
- Hummus—Flavored, mashed chickpeas with tahini and, usually, olive oil
- Loukanika—Sausage
- Tahini—Seasoned paste of crushed raw sesame seeds, used in many dishes

---

In restaurants, the easiest way to have foods low in saturated fat is to select foods low in total fat.

TIPS ON ORDERING LOWER-FAT GREEK FOODS

- For an appetizer, select baked stuffed eggplant, rice mixtures wrapped in grape leaves, or cucumber and yogurt dip rather than fried calamari (squid) or fish roe dip.
- Ask that the olive oil, often added to the top of dips (such as hummus and fish roe dip) and other prepared dishes be omitted.

(continued)

TIPS ON ORDERING LOWER-FAT GREEK FOODS *(continued)*

- When ordering Greek salad, ask that the feta cheese and olives be served on the side so you can control the amount eaten.
- Pita bread, which is often served with appetizers and entrées, is low in fat.
- Choose a chicken pita sandwich instead of a gyro, which contains beef and lamb; yogurt-cucumber sauce can be served on the side so that you can control the amount eaten.
- Since casseroles are made ahead of time, there is no way the fat in them can be reduced. Some restaurants offer small portions of several typical Greek foods on a combination plate, which can be shared with a dinner companion.
- When you order grilled fish or baked chicken, specify that only a small amount of olive oil be used in preparation and added to these dishes before they are served.
- Request that lean meat be used in a shish kebab and that butter not be used to baste it.
- Rizogalo (rice pudding) is lower in fat than baklava (pastry) or galaktoboureko (custard pie). Split a dessert with your dinner companion.

TIPS ON LOWERING SODIUM

- Choose cooked-to-order dishes, such as baked fish, and ask that salt be omitted during food preparation.
- The sodium in casseroles (such as moussaka), spanakopita, dips, and sauces that are made ahead of time, cannot be reduced.
- Feta cheese is higher in sodium than cheddar; it contains about the same amount of sodium as many processed cheeses.

The following table gives you an idea of the calories, fat, saturated fat, and carbohydrate content of selected foods from Greek cuisine. These values are only estimates, and the content of an actual dish may vary, depending on how the chef prepares it.

	Calories	Fat g	Sat. Fat g	Carb. g
APPETIZERS				
Dolmades (8)				
Grape leaves stuffed w/rice, nuts & raisins	290	21	3	25
Hummus (½ c)				
Chickpea dip	240	11	1	29
Kotosoupa avgolemono				
Chicken & rice soup w/egg & lemon	352	14	4	25
Spanakopita (3" x 2")				
Spinach & cheese tart	331	26	14	17
Talattouri (½ c)				
Yogurt & cucumber salad	100	6	1	7
Taramosalata (¼ c)				
Fish roe dip w/onion & olive oil	366	31	5	18
Tsatziki (½ c)				
Yogurt & cucumber dip w/garlic & olive oil	241	14	4	18
ENTRÉES				
Arni psito me patates (6 oz lamb, 3 oz potatoes)				
Roast leg of lamb w/potatoes	694	39	16	20
Giouvetsi				
Baked lamb and pasta (orzo) w/onion & tomato	622	34	16	48
Gyro sandwich				
Beef & lamb in pita bread w/yogurt sauce	257	15	3	19
Keftedes (6)				
Meatballs	293	14	5	14
Moussaka (10 oz)				
Eggplant casserole w/ground meat	321	19	9	17

	Calories	Fat g	Sat. Fat g	Carb. g
Pastitsio (19 oz)				
Baked macaroni & meat pie	953	47	25	78
Psari plaki sto fourno (11 oz)				
Baked fish w/tomatoes, potatoes & olive oil	428	21	3	19
Yemista me lahano (1)				
Cabbage leaves stuffed w/ meat & rice w/egg & lemon sauce	480	27	12	28

ACCOMPANIMENTS

	Calories	Fat g	Sat. Fat g	Carb. g
Bamyes sto fourno (3 oz)				
Baked okra w/olive oil	127	9	1	11
Couscous (1 c)				
w/olive oil	241	5	1	41
Pilaf (1 c)				
Rice w/butter & seasonings	287	5	3	53

BREAD

	Calories	Fat g	Sat. Fat g	Carb. g
Pita (6½" diam)	165	1	0	33

DESSERTS

	Calories	Fat g	Sat. Fat g	Carb. g
Baklava (1)				
Pastry of phyllo, nuts, butter & syrup or honey	176	9	3	22
Galaktoboureko				
Custard-filled phyllo pastry	743	17	10	132
Rizogalo (1 c)				
Creamy rice pudding	357	7	4	62

INDIAN CUISINE

The imaginative use of spices is characteristic of foods originating in India. Some, but not all, Indian dishes are hot from the use of chili peppers. Spices are typically heated in oil; then vegetables, yogurt, cream, and/or meat are added. In Indian cooking, fat is often not drained off after meat or vegetables are cooked.

MENU TERMS THAT INDICATE HIGH FAT

- Ghee—Clarified butter
- Korma—Braised meat with rich yogurt and cream sauce
- Malai—Heavy cream or cream sauce
- Pakora—Deep-fried dough with vegetables

In restaurants, the easiest way to have foods low in saturated fat is to select foods low in total fat.

TIPS ON ORDERING LOWER-FAT INDIAN FOOD

- Select bread and meat cooked in a tandoor (special oven), and request that oil or ghee not be brushed on them.
- Choose a raita or vegetable salad, which is usually served with lemon juice.
- Select a kebab or tandoori entrée (not brushed with fat) instead of a dish with sauce, such as curry; sauces are prepared ahead of time and cannot be specially made with less fat.
- Choose tikka or tandoori meats, since both are low in fat when they are not brushed with fat.

TIP ON LOWERING SODIUM

- Select tandoori or tikka meat as an entrée; they are lower in sodium than entrées with sauce, such as curry.

The following table gives you an idea of the calories, fat, saturated fat, and carbohydrate content of selected foods from Indian cuisine. These values are only estimates, and the content of an actual dish may vary, depending on how the chef prepares it.

	Calories	Fat g	Sat. Fat g	Carb. g
APPETIZERS				
Bhujias (2)				
Onion fritters	99	9	1	4
Gobhi pakoras (2)				
Cauliflower fritters	184	10	1	19
Samosa (1 small)				
Deep-fried pastry filled w/meat	98	7	1	7
Tikkas chicken tandoori (1 thigh)				
Marinated chicken cooked in tandoori				
Not brushed w/fat	111	5	2	0
Brushed w/butter	179	13	6	0
ENTRÉES				
Badsahi badam korma (7 oz)				
Lamb curry w/almonds	494	34	14	10
Chicken chat (4 oz chicken)				
Cold shredded chicken w/ spices on lettuce	353	12	4	18
Gosht do piaza (9 oz)				
Fried lamb & onions simmered in spices & juice	739	66	21	11
Gosht vindaloo (4 oz)				
Beef or lamb w/potatoes in tangy sauce	364	25	11	2
Jhinga masala (8 oz)				
Shrimp in tomato cream sauce	313	26	9	10
Jhinga tandoori (6–8 lg)				
Marinated shrimp cooked in tandoori				
Not brushed w/fat	58	2	0	0
Brushed w/butter	109	7	4	0
Machli masala (10 oz)				
Fish curry	296	11	3	9

	Calories	Fat g	Sat. Fat g	Carb. g
Murgh kari (8 oz)				
Chicken curry	327	20	6	10
Murgh makhani (17 oz)				
Butter chicken	644	47	25	16
Murgh reshmi kabab (3 oz)				
Marinated chicken kebab	224	11	4	0
Rogan josh (8 oz)				
Lamb curry	441	31	7	14
Tandoori chicken (¼ chicken)				
Not brushed w/fat	257	12	3	0
Brushed w/butter after cooking	325	20	8	0

ACCOMPANIMENTS

	Calories	Fat g	Sat. Fat g	Carb. g
Dal maharani (8 oz)				
Creamed lentils w/spices	348	7	1	53
Gobhi matar tamatar (11 oz)				
Cauliflower w/peas & tomatoes	159	8	1	20
Katchumber salad (8 oz)				
Cucumber, onion & tomato salad w/oil & lemon on lettuce leaf	68	3	0	10
Matar paneer (5 oz)				
Fried cheese w/peas	241	18	4	14
Matar pulao (9 oz)				
Rice pilaf w/peas	364	6	4	67
Navarattan curry (9 oz)				
Nine-vegetable curry	259	13	7	34

BREADS

	Calories	Fat g	Sat. Fat g	Carb. g
Chapati or Roti (1)				
Bread cooked on griddle				
Not brushed w/fat	63	2	0	9
Brushed w/oil	103	7	1	9
Nan (1)				
Bread baked in tandoori				
Not brushed w/fat	190	10	5	20
Brushed w/butter	207	12	7	20

	Calories	Fat g	Sat. Fat g	Carb. g
DESSERTS				
Aam malai (4 oz)				
Mango ice cream	287	15	9	35
Kheer (12 oz)				
Indian rice pudding	350	10	6	54
Kulfi (4 oz)				
Ice cream w/pistachios, almonds & rose essence	375	23	12	37
BEVERAGES				
Spiced tea w/whole milk (4 oz)	107	4	3	14
Sweet lassi (3 oz)				
Whole-milk yogurt w/sugar & water	120	2	2	22

ITALIAN CUISINE

Pasta is central to many dishes served in Italian restaurants. The richness of a pasta dish is determined by the type of sauce, amount of cheese, and type of meat in it. Much Italian restaurant cuisine in the United States is similar to dishes of southern Italy, which use tomato sauces instead of the high-fat creamy sauces more common to northern Italian cuisine. Marinara sauce is a popular tomato-based sauce; although usually it is not low in fat because of the oil used in preparation, it is low in saturated fat.

MENU TERMS THAT INDICATE HIGH FAT

- Alfredo—Sauce made with butter, cream, and cheese
- Crema—Cream
- Gelato—Italian ice cream
- Parmigiana—Food is floured, fried, then baked with cheese

In restaurants, the easiest way to have foods low in saturated fat is to select foods low in total fat.

TIPS ON ORDERING LOWER-FAT ITALIAN FOOD

- Choose "cook-to-order" dishes and ask that the oil used be reduced; examples are meat, fish, poultry, and vegetables served with pasta.
- Select red sauces, such as pomodoro and marinara sauce, rather than cream sauces, such as Alfredo sauce.
- Casserole-type dishes (for example, lasagna and cannelloni) contain high-fat ingredients, such as ground meat, sausage, cheese, cream, and butter.
- If fettuccine Alfredo is served with an entrée, request that marinara sauce be substituted for the Alfredo sauce.

TIP ON ORDERING LOWER-SODIUM ITALIAN FOOD

- Choose cooked-to-order dishes and ask that salt be omitted during food preparation.

The following table gives you an idea of the calories, fat, saturated fat, and carbohydrate content of selected foods from Italian cuisine. These values are only estimates, and the content of an actual dish may vary, depending on how the chef prepares it.

	Calories	Fat g	Sat. Fat g	Carb. g
APPETIZERS				
Mixed antipasti (8 oz)				
Ham, fish, cheese & vegetables	314	21	10	8
Bruschetta				
Toasted bread w/tomatoes & olive oil	221	11	2	27
Calamari (8 oz) w/cocktail sauce				
Breaded & fried squid	870	41	9	77
Crab cakes (3½" diam x ½" cakes)				
Fried crab patties (2)	520	33	8	26
Fried mozzarella (4 oz) w/ marinara sauce (½ c)	649	50	21	26
Minestrone (2 c)				
Vegetable soup w/beans	184	4	1	30
Shrimp scampi (8)	135	10	6	0
Stuffed artichoke (1)	577	42	21	39
ENTRÉES				

Some entrées are served with pasta w/tomato sauce (side dish); these values are not included below (see Accompaniments)

	Calories	Fat g	Sat. Fat g	Carb. g
Calzone w/marinara sauce (7" diam folded)				
Pastry w/cheese & meat w/sauce (1 c)	661	24	9	90
Cannelloni (4" long) (2)				
Tube pasta stuffed w/beef & cheese & covered w/sauce	564	27	8	69

	Calories	Fat g	Sat. Fat g	Carb. g
Chicken cacciatore (split chicken breast)				
Sautéed & cooked w/wine	390	17	3	27
Chicken parmigiana (2 split chicken breasts)				
Breaded, fried and baked w/cheese	906	47	23	42
Eggplant parmigiana, (4 pieces, 4" diam)				
Breaded, fried & baked w/cheese	1035	59	29	100
Fettuccine Alfredo (3 c)				
Pasta w/sauce of butter, cream & cheese	1165	59	35	114
Lasagna w/meat (2 pc, ea 3" x 3")				
Pasta baked w/meat sauce & cheese	669	27	15	59
Linguine w/red clam sauce (3 c)	861	23	3	124
Linguine w/white clam sauce (3 c)	1147	38	21	149
Spaghetti (2 c) w/tomato sauce (1 c)	649	11	2	126
Spaghetti (2 c) w/meat sauce (1 c)	766	20	6	112
Spaghetti (2 c) w/meatballs (6 oz or 6 med, 1½" diam) in tomato sauce (1 c)	1140	39	11	145
Spaghetti (2 c) w/Italian sausage (6 oz) & tomato sauce (1 c)	1344	71	22	128
Veal parmigiana (3 cutlets)				
Breaded, fried & baked w/cheese	1152	67	24	58
Veal scallopini (8 oz veal before cooking)				
Breaded and sautéed	607	42	22	7

	Calories	Fat g	Sat. Fat g	Carb. g
ACCOMPANIMENTS				
Italian bread (1 sl, 4½" x 3¼" x ½")	54	1	0	10
Risotto				
Rice w/butter & chicken stock (1 c) as a side dish	239	4	3	45
Spinach, sautéed (1 c)	84	4	2	10
DESSERTS				
Cheesecake (⅛ of 9" diam)	587	42	22	46
Italian ice (½ c)	127	0	0	32
Tiramisu (5" x 4")				
Layered dessert w/espresso-dipped ladyfingers; cream mixture (w/mascarpone cheese and heavy cream); liqueur; chocolate shavings	1161	83	48	84
BEVERAGES				
Cappuccino (1 c)				
Espresso & steamed & frothed milk w/flavored syrup (1 c)	141	6	3	17

JAPANESE CUISINE

Rice is fundamental to Japanese cuisine. Sushi, which is chiefly rice, is probably the most famous Japanese food in the world. Sushi was developed long before the invention of refrigeration, as a means of preventing food from spoiling. Vinegar and seasonings are mixed into freshly cooked rice, which is then pressed or rolled together with vegetables and fresh seafood, often raw. Vinegared rice, topped with raw vegetables, avocado, and/or seafood is often rolled in a nori sheet (dried seaweed) and sliced in bite-size pieces. The trend in American restaurants serving sushi is to include non-traditional foods in rolls. Chefs are now adding fried onions, short ribs, smoked duck, and mozzarella cheese to traditional rolls, which adds calories and saturated fat. Sashimi, raw seafood without the rice, is low in calories and saturated fat.

Japanese dishes typically contain a lot of rice and vegetables, small amounts of meat, fish, and poultry, and little added fat. Seafood, which is significantly lower in fat and saturated fat than meat or poultry, is very important in Japanese cuisine. Most Japanese restaurants don't serve very large portions; however, many people compensate for small portions by over-ordering.

MENU TERMS THAT INDICATE HIGH FAT

- Agedashi—Fried tofu
- Tempura—Seafood and/or vegetables dipped in batter and deep-fried
- Tonkatsu—Breaded and fried pork cutlet

In restaurants, the easiest way to have foods low in saturated fat is to select foods low in total fat.

TIPS ON ORDERING LOWER-FAT JAPANESE FOOD

- Most Japanese sauces do not contain fat, and foods are typically not stir-fried.
- Sashimi and sushi are low in fat; sushi may contain a small egg omelet, raw fish, vegetables, or avocado. (Note: Raw fish can contain parasites, bacteria, and viruses.)
- Select clear soups, such as sumashi wan, which are usually low in fat; some clear soups may contain added egg.
- Avoid fried foods, including anything tempura, dumplings, and spider rolls (fried soft shell crab).
- Choose low-fat entrées, such as yosenabe, teriyaki, shabu shabu, and sukiyaki.
- Some noodle dishes, such as su udon, are low in fat.
- Foods such as oyako domburi (chicken omelet over rice) and chawan mushi (an egg custard dish) are high in cholesterol, since they contain 1 to 2 eggs per serving.

TIPS ON LOWERING SODIUM

- Japanese food is high in sodium from the soy sauce, MSG (monosodium glutamate), and salt used in soups, sauces, marinades, cooking broths, dipping sauces, and salad dressings. Miso is quite high in sodium.
- To reduce your sodium intake, order grilled seafood, chicken, or steaks prepared without marinades, sauces, or added salt.
- Request plain steamed rice. Use dipping sauces sparingly, if at all.
- Sashimi is a low-sodium choice; however, caution is advised in eating raw fish.

The following table gives you an idea of the calories, fat, saturated fat, and carbohydrate content of selected foods from Japanese cuisine. These values are only estimates, and the content of an actual dish may vary, depending on how the chef prepares it.

	Calories	Fat g	Sat. Fat g	Carb. g
SUSHI AND SASHIMI				
Sashimi (3 oz)				
Sliced raw fish				
Raw salmon	121	5	1	0
Raw tuna	122	4	1	0
Sushi (1 roll cut in about 8 pcs)				
California roll				
w/vinegared rice, avocado, crab & mayonnaise	344	10	2	53
Cucumber roll				
w/vinegared rice & cucumber	218	1	0	47
Tuna roll				
w/vinegared rice & raw tuna	249	2	0	45
ENTRÉES				
Gyu niku teriyaki (3 oz)				
Broiled beef w/teriyaki glaze	324	13	5	29
Oyako domburi				
Chicken omelet over rice	507	12	4	68
Shabu shabu (3 oz cooked beef)				
Beef & vegetables cooked in broth at the table	350	19	7	15
Sukiyaki (2 c)				
Meat & vegetables cooked in sauce				
w/beef	555	40	15	12
w/chicken	378	16	4	12
w/pork	458	27	9	12
Tempura (11 oz)				
Deep fried meat & vegetables				
Beef	708	43	11	66
Shrimp	663	39	9	66
Shrimp & tofu	669	52	13	27
Yosenabe (9 oz)				
Seafood & vegetables in broth	156	3	1	13

	Calories	Fat g	Sat. Fat g	Carb. g
MENRUI (NOODLES)				
Su udon				
Hot noodles & broth	287	2	0	55
DIPPING SAUCES				
Ponzu (1 Tbsp)	6	0	0	1
Chirizu, for sashimi (1 Tbsp)	12	0	0	2
Soy sauce (1 Tbsp)	8	0	0	1
Tosa joyu, for sashimi (1 Tbsp)	11	0	0	1

MEXICAN CUISINE

Many of the items found on the menu of a Mexican restaurant differ from the dishes you would find in Mexico; these foods are sometimes termed "TexMex." Some examples of popular TexMex foods are fajitas, nachos, chile con queso, crispy tacos, burritos, and chimichangas. Generally, TexMex foods contain more cheese and have gravy added to them. In Mexico tamales are usually steamed in the corn husk and served with salsa; the TexMex version may be served with gravy.

Entrées served in Mexican restaurants often contain less meat (1 to 2 ounces) than those served in most other types of restaurants. High-fat ingredients, such as cheese, ground meat, and sour cream, are used in many Mexican food dishes. Mexican restaurants differ in the type of fat they use—vegetable oil, partically hydrogenated, or lard—to prepare foods such as refried beans and tostadas.

Corn tortillas and flour tortillas are used as appetizers, in entrées, and as an accompaniment to the meal. Flour tortillas, which often contain lard, provide more than four times the fat of corn tortillas. Corn tortillas contain less than 1 gram of fat unless they are dipped in hot fat for enchiladas or fried, as in tortilla chips, crispy tacos, or tostadas.

MENU TERMS THAT INDICATE HIGH FAT

- Carnitas—Fried pieces of beef or pork
- Chorizo—Highly seasoned sausage of chopped pork
- Quesadilla—Flour tortilla, filled with meat and cheese and grilled
- Refried beans—Beans mashed and cooked with fat, usually lard
- Tamale—Dough made with masa harina, lard or shortening; with ground beef, chicken, or pork filling; wrapped in a corn husk; and steamed
- Tostada or chalupa—Fried tortilla topped with beans, meat, cheese, lettuce, tomato, sour cream, and/or avocado

---

In restaurants, the easiest way to have foods low in saturated fat is to select foods low in total fat.

TIPS ON ORDERING LOWER-FAT MEXICAN FOOD

- When you first sit down, request soft or steamed corn tortillas in place of the tortilla chips usually on the table; dip soft corn tortillas in salsa (hot sauce) as an appetizer instead of ordering nachos (fried tortilla chips, topped with cheese, jalapeño peppers, ground beef, and/or refried beans).
- Request that little or no fat be used in cooking fajitas, which are marinated strips of beef or chicken cooked with onion and bell peppers.
- Choose frijoles a la charra or barracho beans rather than refried beans.
- Request that sour cream and cheese be omitted from dishes or served in side dishes so that you can control the amount used.
- Guacamole (mashed avocado with spices), served as a salad or garnish, is low in saturated fat. The fat it contains is primarily unsaturated.
- Use salsa, which is fat free, as a dressing on chicken fajita salad; request a dish of cilantro or jalapeño peppers for extra zest.
- If you order a salad that is served in a fried tortilla shell, think of the shell as a dish and do not eat it.
- Ask if the restaurant has "off the menu" items, such as grilled fish or chicken breast (usually seasoned with onion, cilantro, and Mexican spices).

TIPS ON LOWERING SODIUM

- Request that cheese not be added to food.
- Request soft or steamed corn tortillas to eat with salsa as an appetizer.
- Order grilled chicken, grilled fish, or fajitas, and ask that salt not be used in preparation; you cannot reduce the sodium in foods already prepared, such as enchiladas, burritos, and tacos.
- Select a fajita salad, and use salsa for the dressing instead of chile con queso or salad dressing.

The following table gives you an idea of the calories, fat, saturated fat, and carbohydrate content of selected foods from Mexican cuisine. These values are only estimates, and the content of an actual dish may vary, depending on how the chef prepares it.

	Calories	Fat g	Sat. Fat g	Carb. g
APPETIZERS				
Chile con queso (½ c)				
Creamy cheese sauce seasoned w/salsa	280	22	11	8
Corn tortilla, soft (6" diam)	58	1	0	12
Flour tortilla (8" diam)	140	3	1	24
Nachos (6)				
Fried tortilla w/toppings				
w/refried beans & cheese	292	17	7	26
w/beef & cheese	260	17	7	9
Tortilla chips (24)	218	11	1	27
ENTRÉES				
Beef fajita meat (8 oz)				
Marinated beef strips	347	18	6	0
Burrito (1)				
Flour tortilla wrapped around assorted fillings				
w/refried beans & cheese	354	15	7	40
Chalupa (2)				
Fried corn tortilla layered w/assorted toppings, cheese, guacamole, lettuce & tomato				
w/chicken, refried beans & cheese	558	29	12	43
w/beef, refried beans & cheese	609	36	15	43
Chicken fajita meat (8 oz)				
Marinated chicken breast strips	225	8	2	0
Chimichanga (2)				
Rolled fried tortilla w/filling				
w/beef	651	44	12	43
w/chicken & cheese	744	50	17	43
w/refried beans & cheese	884	56	20	72

	Calories	Fat g	Sat. Fat g	Carb. g
Enchilada (1)				
Tortilla dipped in hot oil & wrapped around filling w/sauce on top				
w/beef & cheese	679	34	16	55
w/chicken & cheese	590	21	10	55
Fajita salad				
Fried tortilla in shape of bowl filled w/salad (no dressing), meat, guacamole & cheese				
w/grilled chicken, tortilla bowl eaten	812	46	14	59
w/grilled chicken, tortilla bowl not eaten	340	20	8	6
w/grilled beef, tortilla bowl eaten	841	49	16	59
w/grilled beef, tortilla bowl not eaten	369	29	10	6
Tacos, 6½" diam (2)				
Fried tortillas folded in half & filled w/meat, lettuce, tomato & cheese				
w/beef	552	34	13	32
w/chicken	477	25	9	32
ACCOMPANIMENTS				
Frijoles a la charra or Barracho beans (1 c)				
Pinto beans cooked w/bacon	264	4	1	44
Guacamole (½ c)				
Mashed avocado w/onion & spices	187	16	2	13
Ranch style salad dressing (¼ c)	266	27	3	4
Refried beans (1 c)				
Mashed beans fried in fat, usually lard	565	28	11	61
Salsa (½ c)	32	0	0	7
Sour cream (2 Tbsp)	56	6	3	1

	Calories	Fat g	Sat. Fat g	Carb. g
Spanish rice (1 c)				
Rice fried in oil, then cooked w/spices & tomato	240	4	1	46
DESSERTS				
Flan (1)				
Custard w/eggs, milk & sugar, topped w/caramel sauce	264	10	5	38
Sopapilla, 1½" diam (2 sm)				
Dough dropped in hot oil until puffed & golden brown	99	6	2	10

THAI CUISINE

Thai food offers an interesting combination of sharply defined flavors: sweet, hot, sour, salty, and bitter. These flavors are blended in some dishes, while in others one flavor predominates. Entrées, especially curries, are often very hot. Rice is served with most Thai meals to offset the spicy-hot chilies. Most Thai recipes contain sugar, and many incorporate fish sauce, made by fermenting fish with salt. Thai salads, which often combine raw vegetables with shrimp, squid, or beef, are popular.

MENU TERMS THAT INDICATE HIGH FAT

- Coconut milk or coconut cream—Used to prepare curry, sauces, and desserts such as custards
- Peanut sauce—Sauce of coconut milk, fish sauce, sugar, and peanuts, eaten with many Thai dishes

---

In restaurants, the easiest way to have foods low in saturated fat is to select foods low in total fat.

TIPS ON ORDERING LOWER-FAT THAI FOOD

- Order fresh or soft spring rolls rather than fried spring rolls.
- Select stir-fried entrées instead of curry.
- Eat steamed rice rather than fried rice.

TIPS ON LOWERING SODIUM

- Choose cooked-to-order dishes, and ask that MSG and salt be omitted during food preparation.
- Eat steamed rice, which is salt free, instead of fried rice.
- Add very little or no high-sodium fish sauce and soy sauce to food.

The following table gives you an idea of the calories, fat, saturated fat, and carbohydrate content of selected foods from Thai cuisine. These values are only estimates, and the content of an actual dish may vary, depending on how the chef prepares it.

	Calories	Fat g	Sat. Fat g	Carb. g
APPETIZERS				
Gaeng jued woon sen (1 c)				
Glass noodle soup w/pork	197	11	3	12
Gaeng liang (1 c)				
Vegetable soup w/shrimp	115	1	0	16
Po pia taud (6 miniature)				
Fried spring rolls w/pork & shrimp	210	10	2	23
Spring rolls, soft (1)	41	0	0	8
Tom yam goong (1 c)				
Hot & sour shrimp soup	41	0	0	0
SALADS				
Yam nuea (3 oz cooked beef)				
Beef salad	233	13	5	4
Yam po taek (3 oz cooked shrimp, whitefish, squid & clams)				
Seafood salad	147	3	1	10
ENTRÉES				
Gaeng keow wan gai (about 1 c)				
Green curry w/chicken & Thai eggplant	499	34	28	22
Gai pad med mamuang himapan (about 1 c)				
Cashew chicken	408	28	5	13
Gai yang (about 1 c)				
Barbecued chicken	360	17	5	17
Nuea pad kanaa (about 1 c)				
Stir-fried beef w/broccoli	294	18	5	17
Nuea pad prik				
Pepper steak	402	30	9	9

	Calories	Fat g	Sat. Fat g	Carb. g
Pad Thai (about 1 c)				
Stir-fried Thai noodles	484	19	3	62
ACCOMPANIMENTS				
Khao ob sapparod (1 c)				
Rice w/pineapple & coconut milk	688	29	20	102
Khao pad moo (1 c)				
Fried rice w/pork	451	17	4	54
Steamed white rice (1 c)	205	0	0	45
SAUCES AND CONDIMENTS				
Chopped peanuts (2 Tbsp)	106	9	1	3
Peanut sauce (2 Tbsp)	88	7	2	3
DESSERTS				
Khao neeo kaew (1 c)				
Sweet sticky rice w/coconut cream	395	8	7	77
Sangkaya (1 c)				
Thai custard w/egg & coconut cream	508	29	21	55
Ta-Go (1 c)				
Rice pudding w/coconut cream topping	758	42	37	94

VIETNAMESE CUISINE

Vietnamese cuisine reflects the influence of the French, who ruled Vietnam for more than a century; many dishes are similar to Chinese and Thai food, but tend to have less intense, more subtle flavors. Contrasting textures, such as seen in fresh greens and/or crunchy peanuts combined with cooked food, are characteristic of many Vietnamese dishes. Vietnamese food tends to be low in fat, and small amounts of vegetable oil rather than lard are used for stir-frying. All the regional Vietnamese cuisines include fish, shellfish, fresh vegetables, and barbecued dishes.

Nuoc mam is one of the most characteristic ingredients of Vietnamese cuisine. It is commercially prepared by layering fresh anchovies with salt, allowing them to ferment, and draining off the sauce. When lime juice, chilies, sugar, garlic, and vinegar are added to nuoc mam, it is called nuoc cham. Nuoc mam, which is very high in sodium, is used in place of salt at the table and in cooking.

MENU ITEMS THAT INDICATE HIGH FAT

- Curry—Sauce made with coconut milk or heavy cream
- Peanut sauce—Sauce of crushed peanuts, peanut oil, broth, tomato paste, and chili peppers, served with most appetizers and entrées

---

In restaurants the easiest way to have foods low in saturated fat is to select foods low in total fat.

TIPS ON ORDERING LOWER-FAT VIETNAMESE FOOD

- Eat steamed rice rather than fried rice with your entrée.
- When dining with a group, order one less entrée than the number of people and share.
- Select seafood entrées instead of sweet-and-sour or curry dishes
- Eat foods without the addition of peanut sauce.

TIPS ON LOWERING SODIUM

- Choose cooked-to-order dishes, and ask that salt and MSG be omitted during food preparation.
- Eat food without the addition of nuoc mam and muoc cham, which are very high in sodium.
- Eat steamed white rice, which is salt-free, instead of fried rice.

The following table gives you an idea of the calories, fat, saturated fat, and carbohydrate content of selected foods from Vietnamese cuisine. These values are only estimates, and the content of an actual dish may vary, depending on how the chef prepares it.

	Calories	Fat g	Sat. Fat g	Carb. g
APPETIZERS				
Canh chua tom (about 1 c)				
Spicy-and-sour shrimp soup	131	6	1	12
Cha gio (6 miniature rolls)				
Fried spring roll w/pork	224	11	3	23
Thit bo vien				
Steamed meatballs (8 tiny)				
w/chili sauce (2 Tbsp)	97	3	1	4
ENTRÉES				
Bo a lui nuong (3 oz cooked beef)				
Grilled beef wrapped in rice paper w/rice noodles & vegetables	474	14	3	52
Boluc lac (3 oz cooked beef)				
Beef salad served warm over lettuce w/vinaigrette dressing	394	31	5	6
Bun cha (2 skewers w/beef)				
Beef patties cooked on skewer, served w/nuoc cham (not included)	145	9	3	3
Ca hap (4 oz cooked whitefish)				
Steamed whole fish w/bacon	328	18	4	8

	Calories	Fat g	Sat. Fat g	Carb. g
Ca kho to (4 oz cooked halibut)				
Fish simmered in caramel sauce w/pickled bean sprouts, in clay pot	220	2	0	21
Ca-ri ga (about 2 c)				
Chicken curry w/vegetables & coconut milk	488	29	23	34
Heo xao chua ngot				
Sweet and sour pork	423	24	7	21
Muc xao cai chua				
Stir-fried squid	486	14	4	19

SAUCES AND ACCOMPANIMENTS

	Calories	Fat g	Sat. Fat g	Carb. g
Bean sprouts (1 c)	19	0	0	4
Mam nem (¼ c)				
Anchovy & pineapple sauce	63	2	0	10
Nuoc mam				
Fish sauce (1 Tbsp)	8	0	0	1
Peanuts, chopped (1 Tbsp)	53	5	1	2
Peanut sauce (1 Tbsp)				
Peanuts, oil & spices	52	4	1	3
Steamed white rice (1 c)	205	0	0	45

DESSERTS

	Calories	Fat g	Sat. Fat g	Carb. g
Banh dua ca ra men (½ c)				
Coconut flan w/caramel	257	14	9	27
Dau hu nuoc duong (½ c)				
Jellied bean curd w/ginger syrup	346	6	1	65

CHAPTER 4

FAST FOOD

With the fast-paced lifestyle of many Americans, food that can be obtained quickly and easily has become very popular. Although most of the fast foods presently available are high in calories and fat, some selections are not. Those foods that have less saturated fat are the preferred choices.

Soft drinks, juice, milk, regular coffee, and regular tea are basically the same any place they are sold, with only the serving size varying (see Beverages, page 37).

TIPS ON ORDERING LOWER-FAT FAST FOOD

- Order a regular or small hamburger without cheese or bacon instead of a larger hamburger.
- Sliced meat (roast beef or turkey) and grilled chicken sandwiches are usually lower in fat than sandwiches containing ground meat (hamburger and meatball subs), luncheon meat (bologna and salami subs), and/or cheese (grilled cheese, cheeseburger, and meat and cheese subs).
- Choose a salad (without cheese, croutons, or bacon) with "lite" dressing instead of French fries.
- Request pretzels instead of chips.
- Request juice, low-fat milk, or cola (regular or diet) rather than a milkshake.

TIP ON LOWERING SODIUM

- Request lettuce, tomato, and onions on sandwiches instead of condiments that, although low in fat, are high in sodium; these include catsup, mustard, pickles, and steak sauce.

ARBY'S

	Calories	Fat g	Sat. Fat g	Carb. g
SANDWICHES				
Arby-Q	360	11	5	51
Beef 'N Cheddar	440	21	7	44
Big Montana	590	29	14	41
Chicken Bacon 'N Swiss	550	27	7	49
Chicken Breast Fillet	490	24	4	46
Chicken Cordon Bleu	570	29	6	46
French Dip 'N Swiss	320	25	11	56
Giant Roast Beef	450	19	9	41
Grilled Chicken Deluxe	380	12	2	40
Hot Ham 'N Cheese	300	9	4	35
Hot Ham 'N Swiss Melt	270	8	4	35
Junior Roast Beef	270	9	4	34
Market Fresh Low Carbys				
Chicken Caesar Wrap	520	27	7	46
Roast Turkey & Bacon Wrap	710	39	11	48
Southwest Chicken Wrap	550	30	9	45
Ultimate BLT Wrap	650	47	11	48
Market Fresh Sandwiches				
Chicken Salad Sandwich	860	44	6	92
Roast Beef & Swiss Sandwich	780	39	12	74
Roast Ham & Swiss Sandwich	700	31	7	74
Roast Turkey & Swiss Sandwich	720	27	6	74
Roast Turkey, Ranch & Bacon Sandwich	830	38	10	75
Ultimate BLT Sandwich	780	46	9	75
Philly Beef Supreme	450	37	13	59
Regular Roast Beef	320	13	6	34
Roast Chicken Club	470	25	7	39
Super Roast Beef	440	19	7	48
ENTRÉES				
Broccoli 'N Cheddar Baked Potato	460	23	12	56
Chicken Fingers				
4 Pack	640	38	8	42
Combo (4) w/ Curly Fries	1050	60	11	89
Snack (2) w/ Curly Fries	590	34	6	53

	Calories	Fat g	Sat. Fat g	Carb. g
Baked Potato				
Deluxe	570	34	20	50
Plain	200	0	0	46

CONDIMENTS, SAUCES & TOPPINGS

	Calories	Fat g	Sat. Fat g	Carb. g
Arby's Sauce	15	0	0	4
Asian Noodles	71	3	1	8
Au Jus on Side	50	4	1	5
BBQ Dipping Sauce	40	0	0	10
Bronco Berry Sauce	120	0	0	30
Buffalo Dipping Sauce	20	1	0	3
Honey Mustard Dipping Sauce	130	12	2	5
Honey Sauce	60	5	1	3
Horsey Sauce	60	5	1	3
Marinara Sauce	15	0	0	4
Red Ranch Sauce	70	6	1	5
Seasoned Tortilla Strips	61	3	1	10
Sliced Almonds	81	7	0	2
Sour Cream	120	12	7	2
Tangy Southwest Sauce	330	35	5	5
Three Pepper Sauce	20	1	0	3

SALADS

	Calories	Fat g	Sat. Fat g	Carb. g
Asian Sesame Salad	140	1	0	15
Garden Side Salad	35	0	0	7
Martha's Vineyard Salad	250	8	5	23
Santa Fe Salad	520	29	9	40

SALAD DRESSINGS

	Calories	Fat g	Sat. Fat g	Carb. g
Asian Sesame Dressing	190	14	2	15
Buttermilk Ranch Dressing	290	30	5	3
Fat-Free Italian Dressing	30	0	0	7
Light Balsamic Vinaigrette	110	6	1	13
Light Buttermilk Ranch Dressing	100	6	1	12
Raspberry Vinaigrette	172	12	2	16
Santa Fe Ranch Dressing	264	28	4	3

	Calories	Fat g	Sat. Fat g	Carb. g
FRENCH FRIES				
Curly Fries				
Small	340	18	3	39
Medium	410	22	3	47
Large	630	34	5	73
Homestyle Fries				
Small	300	13	2	44
Medium	380	16	3	55
Large	570	24	4	82
SIDE ORDERS				
Jalapeño Bites				
Regular	310	19	7	29
Large	330	37	14	58
Mozzarella Sticks				
Regular	430	23	10	38
Large	850	45	19	76
Onion Petals				
Regular	330	19	3	35
Large	830	48	7	88
Potato Cakes	250	15	2	26
BREAKFAST				
Bacon Biscuit	300	17	5	27
Bacon 'N Egg Croissant	410	26	12	31
Biscuit	230	12	3	26
Ham Biscuit	270	13	4	27
Ham 'N Cheese Croissant	350	19	11	30
Sausage Biscuit	390	27	9	26
Sausage 'N Egg Croissant	510	36	15	31
Scrambled Egg	80	6	2	2
Sourdough Bacon, Egg & Swiss	500	29	10	33
Sourdough Egg 'N Cheese	330	16	6	31
Sourdough Ham, Egg 'N Swiss	450	23	8	33

	Calories	Fat g	Sat. Fat g	Carb. g
DESSERTS				
Apple Turnover (No Icing)	250	10	3	35
Cherry Turnover (No Icing)	250	10	3	35
Icing	130	2	1	29
Gourmet Chocolate Cookie	200	10	6	26
MILKSHAKES, All Flavors				
Regular Shake	510	13	0	83
Large Shake	660	17	0	110

Values are subject to change; however, at the time of printing these were the values published at www.arby.com (5/4/04).

BURGER KING

	Calories	Fat g	Sat. Fat g	Carb. g
HAMBURGERS				
Angus Bacon & Cheese Burger	790	44	19	64
Angus Steak Burger	640	32	12	62
Bacon Cheeseburger	390	20	9	31
Bacon Double Cheeseburger	570	34	17	32
Cheeseburger	350	17	8	31
Double Cheeseburger	530	31	15	32
Double Hamburger	440	23	10	30
Double Whopper	970	61	22	52
w/ Cheese	1060	69	27	53
w/ Cheese w/o Mayo	900	51	24	53
w/o Mayo	810	44	19	52
Hamburger	310	13	5	30
Whopper	700	42	13	52
w/ Cheese	800	49	18	53
w/ Cheese w/o Mayo	640	31	15	53
w/o Mayo	540	24	10	52
Whopper Jr.	390	22	7	31
w/ Cheese	430	26	9	32
w/ Cheese w/o Mayo	350	17	8	32
w/o Mayo	310	13	5	31
SANDWICHES				
BK Fish Filet Sandwich	520	30	8	44
w/o Tartar Sauce	360	13	5	42
BK Veggie Burger	380	16	3	46
w/o Mayo	300	7	2	46
Chicken Sandwich	560	28	6	52
w/o Mayo	460	17	5	52
Chicken Whopper	570	25	5	48
w/o Mayo	410	7	2	48
Spicy TenderCrisp Chicken Sandwich	750	39	7	73
TenderCrisp Chicken Sandwich	810	47	8	72
w/o Mayo	600	23	4	71

	Calories	Fat g	Sat. Fat g	Carb. g
CHICKEN TENDERS				
4 Tenders (Kid's Menu)	170	9	3	10
5 Tenders	210	12	4	13
6 Tenders (Kid's Menu)	250	14	4	15
8 Tenders	340	19	5	20
SAUCES				
Barbecue Dipping Sauce	35	0	0	9
Honey-Flavored Dipping Sauce	90	0	0	23
Honey Mustard Dipping Sauce	90	6	1	9
Ketchup	10	0	0	3
Ranch Dipping Sauce	140	15	3	1
Sweet & Sour Dipping Sauce	40	0	0	10
Zesty Onion Ring Dipping Sauce	150	15	3	3
SALADS				
Fire-Grilled Chicken Caesar Salad w/o Dressing	190	7	3	9
Fire-Grilled Chicken Garden Salad w/o Dressing	210	7	3	12
Fire-Grilled Shrimp Caesar Salad w/o Dressing	180	10	3	9
Fire-Grilled Shrimp Garden Salad w/o Dressing	200	10	3	13
Garden Salad, w/o Dressing	20	0	0	4
SALAD DRESSINGS				
Creamy Garlic Ranch	130	11	2	7
Garden Ranch	120	10	2	7
Hidden Valley Fat-Free Ranch	35	0	0	7
Sweet Onion Vinaigrette	100	8	1	8
Tomato Balsamic Vinaigrette	110	9	1	9
SIDE ORDERS				
Chili	190	8	3	17
French Fries				
Small	230	11	3	29
Medium	360	18	5	46
Large	500	25	7	63
King Size	600	30	8	78

	Calories	Fat g	Sat. Fat g	Carb. g
Onion Rings				
Small	180	9	2	22
Medium	320	16	4	40
Large	480	23	6	60
King Size	550	27	7	70
BREAKFAST				
Croissan'wich				
Bacon, Egg & Cheese	360	22	8	25
Egg & Cheese	320	19	7	24
Ham, Egg & Cheese	360	20	8	25
Sausage & Cheese	420	31	11	23
Sausage, Egg, & Cheese	520	39	14	24
French Toast Sticks (5)	390	20	5	46
Hash Brown Rounds				
Large	390	25	7	38
Small	230	15	4	23
DESSERTS				
Chocolate Chip Cookies	440	16	5	68
Dutch Apple Pie	340	14	3	52
Hershey's Sundae Pie	300	18	10	31
MILKSHAKES				
Chocolate				
Small	410	13	8	65
Medium	600	18	11	97
Large	850	27	17	133
Strawberry				
Small	410	13	8	64
Medium	590	17	11	96
Large	840	26	17	131
Vanilla				
Small	400	15	9	57
Medium	540	20	13	76
Large	800	29	19	113

Values are subject to change; however, at the time of printing these were the values published at www.burgerking.com (5/4/04).

CHICK-FIL-A

	Calories	Fat g	Sat. Fat g	Carb. g
SANDWICHES				
Chargrilled Chicken Sandwich	280	7	2	29
w/o Butter	250	3	1	28
Chargrilled Chicken Club Sandwich w/o Sauce	370	13	5	31
Chargrilled Chicken Deluxe Sandwich	290	7	2	31
Chicken Deluxe Sandwich	420	16	4	39
Chicken Salad Sandwich	350	15	3	32
Chicken Sandwich	410	16	4	38
w/o Butter	380	13	3	37
WRAPS				
Chargrilled Chicken Cool Wrap	380	6	3	54
Chicken Caesar Cool Wrap	460	10	6	52
Spicy Chicken Cool Wrap	380	6	3	52
ENTRÉES				
Chargrilled Chicken (1 Fillet)	100	1	0	1
Chicken (1 Fillet)	230	11	3	10
Chicken Nuggets (8)	260	12	3	12
Chick-N-Strips (4)	290	13	3	14
SOUP & SALADS				
Carrot & Raisin Salad	130	5	1	22
Chargrilled Chicken Garden Salad	180	6	3	9
Chargrilled Chicken Southwest Salad	240	8	4	17
Chick-N-Strips Salad	390	18	5	22
Cole Slaw	210	17	3	14
Side Salad	60	3	2	4
Hearty Breast of Chicken Soup (Regular)	140	4	1	18
SAUCES & TOPPINGS				
Barbecue Sauce	45	0	0	11
Dijon Honey Mustard Sauce	50	5	1	2

	Calories	Fat g	Sat. Fat g	Carb. g
Garlic & Butter Croutons	50	3	0	6
Honey Mustard Sauce	45	0	0	10
Honey-Roasted Sunflower Kernels	80	7	1	3
Polynesian Sauce	110	6	1	13
Tortilla Strips	60	4	1	9
SALAD DRESSINGS				
Blue Cheese	150	16	3	1
Buttermilk Ranch	140	14	2	2
Caesar	160	17	3	1
Fat-Free Dijon Honey Mustard	60	0	0	14
Light Italian	15	1	0	2
Reduced-Fat Raspberry Vinaigrette	80	2	0	15
Spicy	140	14	2	2
Thousand Island	150	14	2	5
FRENCH FRIES				
Waffle Potato Fries				
Small	280	14	5	37
Medium	350	17	4	46
Large	400	19	4	57
BREAKFAST				
Bacon (1 Slice)	30	2	1	0
Bagel, Plain (3 oz)	220	3	0	41
Biscuits				
Plain	260	11	3	38
Bacon, Egg & Cheese	440	24	8	39
Biscuit & Gravy	330	15	4	44
Chicken	420	19	5	44
Sausage	410	23	9	42
Chicken Breakfast Burrito	420	19	6	39
Egg (1 Folded)	90	6	2	1
Fresh Fruit Cup (4 oz)	60	0	0	16
Hashbrowns (3 oz)	260	17	4	25
Sausage (1 Patty)	140	11	6	4

	Calories	Fat g	Sat. Fat g	Carb. g
DESSERTS				
Icedream				
Small Cup	230	6	4	38
Small Cone	160	4	2	28
Lemon Pie	320	10	4	51
Fudge Nut Brownie	330	15	4	45
Cheesecake	340	21	12	30

Values are subject to change; however, at the time of printing these were the values published at www.chick-fil-a.com (5/4/04).

DAIRY QUEEN

	Calories	Fat g	Sat. Fat g	Carb. g
BURGERS				
DQ Homestyle Burgers				
Bacon Double Cheeseburger	610	36	18	31
Cheeseburger	340	17	8	29
Double Cheeseburger	540	31	16	30
Hamburger	290	12	5	29
Ultimate Burger	670	43	19	29
HOT DOGS				
Chili 'n Cheese Dog	330	21	9	22
Hot Dog	240	14	5	19
SANDWICHES & BASKETS				
Breaded Chicken Sandwich	510	27	4	47
Chicken Strip Basket	1000	50	13	102
Grilled Chicken Sandwich	340	16	3	26
SALADS				
Crispy Chicken Salad w/o Dressing	350	20	6	21
Grilled Chicken Salad w/o Dressing	240	10	5	12
Side Salad w/o Dressing	60	3	2	6
SALAD DRESSINGS				
DQ Blue Cheese	210	20	4	4
DQ Honey Mustard	260	21	4	18
DQ Ranch	310	33	5	3
Fat-Free Buttermilk Ranch	30	0	0	6
Fat-Free Red French	40	0	0	10
Fat-Free Honey Mustard	50	0	0	13
Fat-Free Italian	10	0	0	3
Fat-Free Ranch	60	0	0	13
Fat-Free Thousand Island	60	0	0	16
Reduced Calorie Buttermilk	140	13	2	5
Wish-Bone Fat-Free Italian	25	0	0	6

	Calories	Fat g	Sat. Fat g	Carb. g
FRENCH FRIES & ONION RINGS				
French Fries				
Small	300	12	3	45
Medium	380	15	3	56
Large	480	19	4	72
Onion Rings	470	30	6	45
BLIZZARDS				
Banana Split Blizzard				
Small	460	14	9	73
Medium	580	17	11	97
Large	810	23	15	134
Chocolate Chip Cookie Dough Blizzard				
Small	720	28	14	105
Medium	1030	40	20	150
Large	1320	52	26	193
Oreo Cookies Blizzard				
Small	570	21	10	83
Medium	700	26	12	103
Large	1010	37	18	148
FROZEN DESSERTS				
Banana Split	510	12	8	96
Brownie Earthquake	740	27	16	112
Buster Bar	450	28	12	41
Chocolate Dilly Bar	210	13	7	21
DQ Frozen 8" Round Cake	370	13	8	56
DQ Fudge Bar, No Sugar Added	50	0	0	13
DQ Sandwich	200	6	3	31
DQ Vanilla Orange Bar, No Sugar Added	60	0	0	17
Lemon DQ Freez'r (½ c)	80	0	0	20
Peanut Buster Parfait	730	31	17	99
Pecan Praline Parfait	720	29	11	105
Starkiss	80	0	0	21
Strawberry Shortcake	430	14	9	70
Triple Chocolate Utopia	770	39	17	96

	Calories	Fat g	Sat. Fat g	Carb. g
ICE CREAM				
DQ Chocolate Soft Serve (½ c)	150	5	4	22
DQ Vanilla Soft Serve (½ c)	140	5	3	22
Chocolate Cone				
Small	240	8	5	37
Medium	340	11	7	53
Dipped Cone				
Small	340	17	9	42
Medium	490	24	13	59
Large	710	36	17	85
Vanilla Cone				
Small	230	7	5	38
Medium	330	9	6	53
Large	480	15	9	76
SUNDAES				
Chocolate Sundae				
Small	280	7	5	49
Medium	400	10	6	71
Large	580	15	10	100
Strawberry Sundae				
Small	240	7	5	40
Medium	340	9	6	58
Large	500	15	9	83
MILKSHAKES, MALTS & MISTY				
Chocolate Malt				
Small	640	16	11	111
Medium	870	22	14	153
Large	1320	35	22	222
Chocolate Shake				
Small	560	15	10	93
Medium	760	20	13	129
Large	1140	33	21	186
Misty Slush				
Small	220	0	0	56
Medium	290	0	0	74

Values are subject to change; however, at the time of printing these were the values published at www.dairyqueen.com (11/3/04).

DOMINO'S PIZZA

	Calories	Fat g	Sat. Fat g	Carb. g
12" CLASSIC HAND TOSSED (⅛ of pizza)				
America's Favorite Feast	257	12	5	29
Bacon Cheeseburger Feast	273	13	6	28
Barbecue Feast	252	10	5	31
Beef	225	9	4	28
Cheese	186	5	2	28
Deluxe Feast	234	10	4	29
ExtravaganZZa Feast	289	14	6	30
Green Pepper, Onion & Mushroom	191	6	2	29
Ham	198	6	3	28
Ham & Pineapple	200	6	3	29
Hawaiian Feast	223	8	4	30
MeatZZa Feast	281	14	6	29
Pepperoni	223	9	4	28
Pepperoni & Sausage	255	12	5	28
Pepperoni Feast	265	13	5	28
Sausage	231	10	4	28
Vegi Feast	218	8	4	29
12" ULTIMATE DEEP DISH (⅛ of pizza)				
America's Favorite Feast	309	17	6	29
Bacon Cheeseburger Feast	325	19	7	28
Barbecue Feast	304	15	6	32
Beef	277	15	5	28
Cheese	238	11	4	28
Deluxe Feast	287	15	5	29
ExtravaganZZa Feast	341	20	7	30
Green Pepper, Onion & Mushroom	244	11	4	30
Ham	250	12	4	28
Ham & Pineapple	252	12	4	30
Hawaiian Feast	275	13	5	30
MeatZZA Feast	333	19	7	29
Pepperoni	275	14	5	28
Pepperoni & Sausage	307	17	6	29
Pepperoni Feast	317	18	7	29
Sausage	283	15	5	29
Vegi Feast	270	14	4	30

	Calories	Fat g	Sat. Fat g	Carb. g
12″ CRUNCHY THIN CRUST (⅛ of pizza)				
America's Favorite Feast	208	14	5	15
Bacon Cheeseburger Feast	224	15	6	14
Barbecue Feast	203	12	5	17
Beef	175	11	4	14
Cheese	137	7	3	14
Deluxe Feast	185	12	4	15
ExtravaganZZa Feast	240	16	6	16
Green Pepper, Onion & Mushroom	142	8	3	15
Ham	148	8	3	14
Ham & Pineapple	150	8	3	15
Hawaiian Feast	174	10	4	16
MeatZZa Feast	232	15	6	15
Pepperoni	174	11	4	14
Pepperoni & Sausage	206	14	5	14
Pepperoni Feast	216	14	6	14
Sausage	181	11	4	14
Vegi Feast	168	10	4	15
14″ CLASSIC HAND TOSSED (⅛ of pizza)				
America's Favorite Feast	353	16	6	39
Bacon Cheeseburger Feast	379	18	8	38
Barbecue Feast	344	14	6	43
Beef Classic	312	13	5	38
Cheese	256	8	3	38
Deluxe Feast Classic	316	13	5	39
ExtravaganZZa Feast	388	19	8	40
Green Pepper, Onion & Mushroom	263	8	3	39
Ham	272	9	4	38
Ham & Pineapple	275	9	4	40
Hawaiian Feast	309	11	5	41
MeatZZa Feast	378	18	8	39
Pepperoni	305	12	3	38
Pepperoni & Sausage	350	16	6	39
Pepperoni Feast	363	17	7	39
Sausage	320	14	5	39
Vegi Feast	300	11	5	40

Domino's Pizza

	Calories	Fat g	Sat. Fat g	Carb. g
14" ULTIMATE DEEP DISH (⅛ of pizza)				
America's Favorite Feast	433	24	8	42
Bacon Cheeseburger Feast	459	26	10	41
Barbecue Feast	424	21	8	46
Beef	392	20	7	41
Cheese	336	15	5	41
Deluxe Feast	396	20	7	42
ExtravaganZZa Feast	468	26	10	43
Green Pepper, Onion & Mushroom	343	15	5	42
Ham	352	16	6	41
Ham & Pineapple	355	16	6	42
Hawaiian Feast	389	18	7	43
MeatZZa Feast	458	25	10	42
Pepperoni	385	20	7	41
Pepperoni & Sausage	430	23	8	41
Pepperoni Feast	443	24	9	42
Sausage	400	21	7	42
Vegi Feast	380	18	7	43
14" CRUNCHY THIN CRUST (⅛ of pizza)				
America's Favorite Feast	285	19	7	20
Bacon Cheeseburger Feast	311	21	9	19
Barbecue Feast	276	16	7	24
Beef	243	15	6	19
Cheese	188	10	4	19
Deluxe Feast	248	15	6	20
ExtravaganZZa Feast	320	21	8	21
Green Pepper, Onion & Mushroom	201	8	4	21
Ham	204	8	4	19
Ham & Pineapple	207	8	4	21
Hawaiian Feast	240	13	5	21
MeatZZa Feast	310	20	8	20
Pepperoni	237	15	6	19
Pepperoni & Sausage	282	19	7	19
Pepperoni Feast	295	19	8	20
Sausage	252	16	6	20
Vegi Feast	231	14	4	21

	Calories	Fat g	Sat. Fat g	Carb. g
SIDE ORDERS				
Barbecue Buffalo Wings (1)	50	3	1	2
Buffalo Chicken Kickers (1)	47	2	1	3
Hot Buffalo Wings (1)	45	3	1	1
Breadstick (1)	115	6	1	12
Cheesy Bread (1)	123	7	2	13
Cinna Stix (1)	123	6	1	15
Sweet Icing (1 container)	250	3	3	57
SAUCES				
Blue Cheese Dipping Sauce	223	24	4	2
Hot Dipping Sauce	15	0	0	4
Ranch Dipping Sauce	197	21	3	2
Garlic Sauce	440	49	10	0
Marinara Dipping Sauce	25	0	0	5

Values are subject to change; however, at the time of printing these were the values published at www.dominos.com (6/4/04).

DUNKIN' DONUTS

	Calories	Fat g	Sat. Fat g	Carb. g
DONUTS				
Apple Crumb	230	10	3	34
Apple N' Spice	200	8	2	29
Bavarian Kreme	210	9	2	30
Black Raspberry	210	8	2	32
Blueberry Cake	290	16	4	35
Blueberry Crumb	240	10	3	36
Boston Kreme	240	9	2	36
Bow Tie	300	17	4	34
Chocolate Coconut Cake	300	19	6	31
Chocolate Frosted Cake	360	20	5	40
Chocolate Frosted	200	9	2	29
Chocolate Glazed Cake	290	16	4	33
Chocolate Kreme Filled	270	13	3	35
Cinnamon Cake	330	20	5	34
Double Chocolate Cake	310	17	4	37
French Cruller	150	8	2	17
Frosted Lemon Cake	240	14	4	28
Glazed Cake	350	19	5	41
Glazed Yeast	180	8	2	25
Glazed Lemon Cake	240	14	4	28
Jelly Filled	210	8	2	32
Lemon Burst	300	14	5	35
Maple Frosted	210	9	2	30
Marble Frosted	200	9	2	29
Old Fashioned Cake	300	19	5	28
Powdered Cake	330	19	5	36
Strawberry	210	8	2	32
Strawberry Frosted	210	9	2	30
Sugar Raised	170	8	2	22
Vanilla Kreme Filled	270	13	3	36
Whole Wheat Glazed Cake	310	19	4	32
SPECIALTIES				
Apple Fritter	300	14	3	41
Chocolate Frosted Coffee Roll	290	15	3	36
Chocolate Iced Bismarck	340	15	4	50
Coffee Roll	270	14	3	33

	Calories	Fat g	Sat. Fat g	Carb. g
Éclair	270	11	3	39
Glazed Fritter	260	14	3	31
Maple Frosted Coffee Roll	290	14	3	36
Vanilla Frosted Coffee Roll	290	14	3	36
STICKS				
Cinnamon Cake	450	30	7	42
Glazed Cake	490	29	7	51
Glazed Chocolate Cake	470	29	7	49
Jelly	530	29	7	61
Plain Cake	420	29	7	35
Powdered Cake	450	29	7	42
MUNCHKINS				
Cinnamon Cake (4)	270	15	4	31
Glazed Cake (3)	280	13	3	38
Glazed Chocolate Cake (3)	200	10	2	26
Glazed Yeast (5)	200	13	2	27
Jelly-Filled Yeast (5)	210	9	2	30
Lemon Filled Yeast (4)	170	8	2	23
Plain Cake (4)	270	16	4	27
Powdered Cake (4)	270	14	4	31
Sugar Raised Yeast (7)	220	12	3	26
SCONES				
Maple Walnut	470	22	5	62
Raspberry White Chocolate	450	22	7	59
HOT BEVERAGES (10 oz)				
Cappuccino	80	5	3	7
w/ Sugar	130	5	3	21
w/ Soy Milk	70	3	0	6
Caramel Swirl Latte	230	6	4	36
w/ Soy Milk	210	4	0	34
Coffee	15	0	0	3
Dunkaccino	230	10	3	35
Hot Chocolate	220	8	2	38
Latte	120	6	4	10
w/ Sugar	160	6	4	22
w/ Soy Milk	90	4	0	8

	Calories	Fat g	Sat. Fat g	Carb. g
Mocha Swirl Latte	230	7	4	37
w/ Soy Milk	210	5	1	35

ICED BEVERAGES (16 oz)

	Calories	Fat g	Sat. Fat g	Carb. g
Coffee Coolatta				
w/ Skim Milk	170	0	0	41
w/ 2% Milk	190	2	2	41
w/ Whole Milk	210	4	3	42
w/ Cream	350	22	14	40
Iced Caramel Swirl Latte	240	7	4	37
w/ Soy Milk	210	4	0	34
Iced Latte	120	7	4	11
w/ Soy Milk	90	4	0	8
Iced Mocha Swirl Latte	240	8	5	38
w/ Soy Milk	210	5	1	35
Lemonade Coolata	240	0	0	59
Orange Mango Fruit Coolatta	270	0	0	66
Strawberry Fruit Coolatta	290	0	0	72
Vanilla Bean Coolatta	440	17	15	70
Vanilla Chai	230	8	6	40

Values are subject to change; however, at the time of printing these were the values published at www.dunkindonuts.com (7/4/04).

EINSTEIN BROS BAGELS

	Calories	Fat g	Sat. Fat g	Carb. g
BAGELS				
Asiago Cheese Bagel	360	3	2	71
Chocolate Chip Bagel	370	3	2	76
Chopped Garlic Bagel	380	3	1	79
Chopped Onion Bagel	330	1	0	71
Cinnamon Raisin Swirl Bagel	350	1	0	78
Cinnamon Sugar Bagel	330	1	0	74
Cinnamon Sugar Bagel Chicago Style	500	21	5	72
Cranberry Bagel	350	1	0	78
Dark Pumpernickel Bagel	320	1	0	68
Egg Bagel	340	3	1	69
Everything Bagel	340	2	0	75
Honey Whole Wheat Bagel	320	1	0	71
Lower Carb 9-Grain Bagel	210	4	1	28
Lower Carb 9-Grain Plain Cream Cheese Bagel	310	13	7	29
Mango Bagel	360	1	0	80
Marble Rye Bagel	340	2	0	73
Nutty Banana Bagel	360	3	1	74
Plain Bagel	320	1	0	71
Poppy Dip'd Bagel	350	2	0	74
Potato Bagel	350	5	1	69
Power Bagel	410	5	1	81
Power Bagel w/ Peanut Butter	750	34	6	92
Pumpkin Bagel	330	2	0	72
Roasted Red Pepper & Pesto Bagel	410	7	4	73
Salt Bagel	330	1	0	73
Sesame Dip'd Bagel	380	5	1	75
Six-Cheese Bagel	390	6	3	72
Spicy Nacho Bagel	450	9	5	77
Spinach Florentine Bagel	410	7	4	72
Sun-Dried Tomato Bagel	320	1	0	69
Wild Blueberry Bagel	350	1	0	77
CREAM CHEESE, Whipped				
Blueberry	70	5	4	6
Cappuccino	70	5	3	5

	Calories	Fat g	Sat. Fat g	Carb. g
Garden Vegetable	60	5	4	3
Honey Almond	70	5	3	6
Jalapeño Salsa	60	5	3	3
Maple Raisin & Walnut	60	5	4	4
Onion & Chive	70	6	4	3
Plain	70	7	5	1
Reduced Fat	60	5	4	2
Pumpkin	100	8	6	6
Smoked Salmon	60	6	4	2
Strawberry	70	5	4	5
Sun Dried Tomato & Basil	60	5	4	2
SPREADS/SHMEARS				
Butter & Margarine Spread	60	7	2	0
Feta Pinenut Spread	60	5	3	2
Grape Spread	75	0	0	19
Honey Butter	90	9	4	4
Hummus	110	7	1	9
Peanut Butter, Creamy	190	15	2	8
Peppercorn Spread	100	10	3	2
Spicy Roasted Tomato Spread	140	14	2	3
Strawberry Spread	75	0	0	19
SANDWICHES				
100% Albacore Tuna on Artisan Wheat	400	9	1	49
Bagel Dog on 9-Grain Bagel	560	33	13	35
Black Forest Ham on Challah	620	23	8	65
Cali Club Panini	990	56	19	71
Club Mex on Challah	920	53	17	65
Cobbie on Challah	810	44	16	65
Einstein Club on Rustic White	840	44	12	55
Ham & Cheese Panini	640	23	10	68
Italian Chicken Panini	690	27	10	68
Mediterranean Hummus & Feta on Ciabatta	450	10	4	77
New York Lox & Bagel	660	27	19	79
Roasted Turkey on Artisan Wheat	610	28	10	51

	Calories	Fat g	Sat. Fat g	Carb. g
Tasty Turkey on 9-Grain Bagel	490	18	10	40
Tasty Turkey on Asiago Bagel	630	19	11	83
Tuna Salad on 9-Grain Bagel	360	9	2	34
Turkey Deli on 9-Grain Bagel	330	6	2	32
Veg Out on Sesame Seed Bagel	500	13	7	82
CONDIMENTS				
Ancho Lime Mayo	50	5	1	1
Ancho Lime Salsa	20	1	0	3
Deli Mustard	4	0	0	0
French Dijon Mustard	10	0	0	0
Gorgonzola Mayo	50	5	3	1
Grained Dijon Mustard	5	0	0	0
Honey Mustard	15	0	0	2

Values are subject to change; however, at the time of printing these were the values published at www.einsteinbros.com (7/4/04).

FAZOLI'S ITALIAN RESTAURANTS

	Calories	Fat g	Sat. Fat g	Carb. g
ENTRÉES				
Lasagna				
Broccoli Six Layer	680	28	12	38
Six Layer w/ Meat Sauce	620	23	11	33
Twice Baked	890	43	24	36
Pasta				
Baked Chicken Parmesan	760	16	4	110
Broccoli Fettuccine Alfredo				
Small	590	17	4	89
Regular	840	22	6	129
Cheese Ravioli w/ Marinara	580	15	7	85
w/ Meat Sauce	610	16	8	85
Chicken Broccoli Bake	560	27	14	13
Classic Meaty Ziti				
Small	500	24	14	37
Regular	760	37	21	58
Fettuccine Alfredo				
Small	500	11	4	81
Regular	740	15	5	122
Garden Style Chicken Penne	830	28	2	100
Peppery Chicken Alfredo				
Small	570	12	4	81
Regular	820	17	5	122
Roasted Garlic Alfredo	710	17	5	101
Spicy Marinara Penne				
w/ Chicken	990	13	2	178
Tuscan Chicken Bake	660	29	14	53
Twice Baked Ziti w/ Meat Sauce	1340	81	49	60
Samplers				
Classic Sampler w/ 6 Layer Lasagna	790	18	8	99
Ultimate Sampler Platter	1010	29	13	116
Spaghetti				
Baked Spaghetti Parmesan	700	25	13	76
Baked Spaghetti w/ Meatballs	970	42	22	91

	Calories	Fat g	Sat. Fat g	Carb. g
Spaghetti w/ Marinara Sauce				
Small	440	2	0	84
Regular	650	3	0	126
Spaghetti w/ Meatballs				
Small	690	20	8	91
Regular	980	27	10	135
Spaghetti w/ Meat Sauce				
Small	460	4	2	84
Regular	690	6	2	125

PIZZA

	Calories	Fat g	Sat. Fat g	Carb. g
Brick-Oven Style (9 x 9" Square)				
Italian Meat	970	46	19	92
Mediterranean	890	43	17	85
Pepperoni	870	39	16	89
Spicy Southwest Chicken	830	32	13	89
Ultimate Cheese	800	32	16	89
Kids Pizza (6" Round)				
Cheese	380	15	8	43
Pepperoni	450	21	10	43

SANDWICHES

	Calories	Fat g	Sat. Fat g	Carb. g
Panini				
Chicken Caesar Club	740	41	16	47
Chicken Pesto	580	28	8	50
Four Cheese & Tomato	820	52	21	51
Grilled Chicken	380	7	3	50
Smoked Turkey	710	40	12	51
Submarino				
Club	1040	44	12	117
Ham & Swiss	980	38	10	117
Meatball	1110	44	20	124
Original	1390	78	22	116
Turkey	940	36	9	114

SALADS

	Calories	Fat g	Sat. Fat g	Carb. g
Caesar Side	110	5	2	12
Chicken & Pasta Caesar	520	34	7	27
Chicken Caesar	190	6	2	14

	Calories	Fat g	Sat. Fat g	Carb. g
Garden	25	0	0	4
Grilled Chicken	110	2	0	6
Italian Market	620	41	13	32
Side Pasta	240	14	4	22
			2	
SALAD DRESSINGS				
Honey French	150	12	2	9
House Italian	110	9	2	5
Ranch	150	17	3	1
Reduced Calorie Italian	50	5	1	3
Thousand Island	130	13	2	4
SOUP				
Minestrone	90	0	0	19
BREADSTICKS				
Breadstick (1)	140	6	1	18
Breadstick, Dry (1)	100	2	0	18
DESSERTS				
Cheesecake				
Plain	290	22	14	17
Turtle	420	34	17	24
Freezi				
Strawberry	510	6	6	115
Strawberry Banana	530	6	6	118
Triple Berry	520	6	6	116
Fresh Baked Chocolate				
Chunk Cookie	590	28	12	77
Lemon Ice	190	0	0	45
Strawberry Topping	35	0	0	8

Values are subject to change; however, at the time of printing these were the values published at www.fazolis.com (11/8/04).

JAMBA JUICE

	Calories	Fat g	Sat. Fat g	Carb. g
SMOOTHIES (24 oz)				
Aloha Pineapple	470	2	1	89
Banana Berry	470	2	1	112
Berry Lime Sublime	450	2	1	104
Caribbean Passion	440	2	1	102
Chocolate Moo'd	690	8	5	142
Citrus Squeeze	450	2	1	93
Coldbuster	430	3	1	100
Cranberry Craze	420	2	1	97
Endless Lime	610	2	1	140
Jamba Powerboost	440	2	0	103
Kiwi Berry Burner	470	0	0	112
Lime It Up!	530	2	1	126
Mango-A-Go-Go	500	2	1	117
Orange Berry Blitz	410	3	1	94
Orange Dream Machine	540	3	1	112
Orange-A-Peel	440	1	0	102
Peach Pleasure	460	2	1	108
Peanut Butter Moo'd	860	21	5	145
Peenya Kowlada	650	5	4	118
Protein Berry Pizzazz	440	2	0	92
Razzmatazz	480	2	1	112
Strawberries Wild	450	0	0	105
Strawberry Tsunami	530	2	1	128
LIGHT SMOOTHIES (24 oz)				
Berry Fulfilling	290	1	0	62
Mango Mantra	310	1	0	71
Orange Divine	280	1	0	63
Strawberry Nirvana	280	1	0	64
JUICES (24 oz)				
Carrot Juice	150	1	0	34
Lemonade	450	0	0	112
Mango Lemonade	420	0	0	107
Orange Juice	330	2	1	77
Orange/Banana Juice	350	2	0	84
Orange/Carrot Juice	240	2	0	56

	Calories	Fat g	Sat. Fat g	Carb. g
Vibrant C Juice	380	1	0	92
Wheatgrass Juice (2 oz)	15	0	0	2
BAKERY				
Apple Cinnamon Pretzel	410	5	0	78
Grin N' Carrot	250	10	1	36
Honey Berry Bran	320	12	2	48
Lemon Poppyseed Bundt	300	12	2	44
Pizza Protein Stick	230	6	2	33
Sourdough Parmesan Pretzel	460	11	2	75

Values are subject to change; however, at the time of printing these were the values published at www.jambajuice.com (6/4/04).

KENTUCKY FRIED CHICKEN

	Calories	Fat g	Sat. Fat g	Carb. g
ENTRÉES				
Chicken Pot Pie	770	40	15	70
Crispy Strips (3)	400	24	5	17
Extra Crispy Chicken				
Breast	460	28	8	19
Drumstick	160	10	3	5
Thigh	370	26	7	12
Whole Wing	190	11	4	10
Honey BBQ Boneless Wings (6)				
w/ Sauce	600	28	5	49
Honey BBQ Wings w/ Sauce	540	33	7	36
Hot & Spicy Chicken				
Breast	460	27	8	20
Drumstick	150	9	3	4
Thigh	400	28	8	14
Whole Wing	180	11	3	9
Hot Wings (6)	450	29	6	23
Original Recipe Chicken				
Breast	380	19	6	11
w/o Skin or Breading	140	3	1	0
Drumstick	140	8	2	4
Thigh	360	25	7	12
Whole Wing	150	12	3	5
Oven Roasted Strips Meal (3 Strips, Green Ceans, Seasoned Rice)	420	7	3	50
Popcorn Chicken				
Kids	270	18	4	18
Individual	430	29	6	26
Large	660	44	10	37
SANDWICHES				
Honey BBQ Flavored				
Sandwich w/ Sauce	300	6	2	41
Original Recipe Sandwich				
w/ Sauce	450	27	6	22
w/o Sauce	320	13	4	21

	Calories	Fat g	Sat. Fat g	Carb. g
Tender Roast Sandwich				
w/ Sauce	390	19	4	24
w/o Sauce	260	5	2	23
Triple Crunch Sandwich				
w/ Sauce	670	40	8	42
w/o Sauce	540	26	6	41
Twister Sandwich	670	38	7	55
Zinger Sandwich				
w/ Sauce	680	41	8	42
w/o Sauce	540	26	6	41
SIDE ORDERS				
BBQ Baked Beans	230	1	1	46
Biscuit	190	10	2	23
Cole Slaw	190	11	2	22
Corn on the Cob				
3"	70	2	1	13
6"	150	3	1	26
Green Beans	50	2	1	5
Mac & Cheese	130	6	2	15
Mashed Potatoes				
w/ Gravy	120	4	1	18
w/o Gravy	110	4	1	16
Potato Salad	180	9	2	22
Potato Wedges	240	12	3	30
DESSERTS				
Apple Pie	270	9	2	45
Cherry Cheesecake Parfait	300	11	5	48
Double Chocolate Chip Cake	400	29	5	31
Lemon Meringue Pie	310	11	5	47
Lil' Bucket				
Fudge Brownie	270	9	4	44
Lemon Crème	400	14	7	65
Chocolate Crème	270	13	8	37
Strawberry Shortcake	200	6	4	34
Pecan Pie	370	15	3	55
Strawberry Crème Pie	270	12	7	37

Values are subject to change; however, at the time of printing these were the values published at www.kfc.com (5/4/04).

KRISPY KREME DOUGHNUTS

	Calories	Fat g	Sat. Fat g	Carb. g
YEAST DOUGHNUTS				
Caramel Kreme Crunch	350	19	5	43
Chocolate Iced				
Custard Filled	300	17	4	35
Iced Glazed	250	12	3	33
Kreme Filled	350	20	5	38
w/ Sprinkles	260	12	3	38
Cinnamon Apple Filled	290	16	4	32
Cinnamon Bun	260	16	4	28
Cinnamon Twist	230	9	3	33
Dulce De Leche	290	18	5	30
Glazed				
Cherry Filled	290		4	36
Cinnamon	210	12	3	24
Kreme Filled	340	20	5	38
Lemon Filled	290	16	4	35
Original Glazed	200	12	3	22
Raspberry Filled	300	16	4	39
Key Lime Pie	320	17	5	40
Maple Iced Glazed	240	12	3	32
New York Cheesecake	320	19	5	35
Powdered				
Blueberry Filled	290	16	4	33
Strawberry Filled	290	16	4	33
Sugar Doughnut	200	12	3	21
CAKE DOUGHNUTS				
Chocolate Glazed Cruller	290	15	4	37
Chocolate Iced	270	14	3	36
Glazed				
Blueberry	330	17	4	43
Chocolate	300	15	4	41
Cruller	240	14	4	26
Pumpkin Spice	340	18	5	42
Sour Cream	340	18	5	42
Powdered	260	14	3	37
Traditional	230	13	3	25

Values are subject to change; however, at the time of printing these were the values published at www.krispykreme.com (7/4/04).

LONG JOHN SILVER'S

	Calories	Fat g	Sat. Fat g	Carb. g
ENTRÉES				
Baked Cod	120	5	1	0
Battered Chicken Plank	140	8	3	9
Battered Fish	230	13	4	16
Battered Shrimp	45	3	1	3
Breaded Clams	240	13	2	22
Clam Strips	240	13	2	22
Crunchy Shrimp Basket (21 pc)	340	19	5	32
Lobster Crab Cake	170	9	2	16
SANDWICHES				
Chicken Sandwich	360	15	4	41
Fish Sandwich				
w/ Tarter Sauce	440	20	5	48
w/o Tarter Sauce	390	16	5	45
Ultimate Fish Sandwich				
w/ Tarter Sauce	500	25	8	48
w/o Tarter Sauce	460	21	1	46
SOUP				
Clam Chowder Bowl	220	10	4	23
SALADS				
Crispy Chicken Salad	580	33	9	43
Shrimp & Seafood Salad	330	15	5	30
SALAD DRESSINGS				
Fat-Free French	50	0	0	12
Garden Ranch	230	24	4	2
Lite Italian	20	1	0	3
Thousand Island	220	21	4	7
SIDE ORDERS				
Cheesesticks (3)	140	8	2	12
Cole Slaw	200	15	3	15
Corn Cobbette	90	3	1	14
Crumblies	170	12	3	14

	Calories	Fat g	Sat. Fat g	Carb. g
French Fries				
Regular	230	10	3	34
Large	390	17	4	56
Hushpuppies	60	3	1	9
Rice	180	4	1	34
CONDIMENTS				
Honey Mustard Sauce	20	0	0	5
Ketchup	10	0	0	2
Malt Vinegar	0	0	0	0
Shrimp Sauce	15	0	0	3
Sweet 'n Sour Sauce	20	0	0	5
Tartar Sauce	40	4	1	2
DESSERTS				
Chocolate Crème Pie	310	22	14	24
Pecan Pie	370	15	3	55
Pineapple Crème Pie	290	13	7	39

Values are subject to change; however, at the time of printing these were the values published at www.ljsilvers.com (11/9/04).

McDONALD'S

	Calories	Fat g	Sat. Fat g	Carb. g
SANDWICHES				
Big Mac	600	33	11	50
Big 'N Tasty				
w/ Cheese	590	36	12	39
w/o Cheese	540	32	10	38
Cheeseburger	330	14	6	36
Chicken McGrill	400	16	3	37
Crispy Chicken	510	26	5	47
Double Quarter Pounder w/ Cheese	770	47	20	39
Double Cheeseburger	490	26	12	38
Filet-O-Fish	410	20	4	41
Hamburger	280	10	4	36
Hot 'N Spicy McChicken	450	26	5	40
McChicken	430	23	5	41
Quarter Pounder				
w/ Cheese	540	29	13	39
w/o Cheese	430	21	8	38
McNUGGETS & SAUCES				
4 McNuggets	170	10	2	10
6 McNuggets	250	15	3	15
10 McNuggets	420	24	5	26
20 McNuggets	840	49	11	51
Barbeque Sauce	45	0	0	10
Honey	45	0	0	12
Hot Mustard Sauce	60	4	0	7
Sweet 'N Sour Sauce	50	0	0	11
FRENCH FRIES				
Small	220	11	2	28
Medium	350	17	3	44
Large	520	25	5	66
HAPPY MEALS				
Cheeseburger, Fries & Milk	660	28	10	77
Hamburger, Fries & Milk	610	23	7	76
McNuggets (4), Fries & Milk	500	23	6	51

	Calories	Fat g	Sat. Fat g	Carb. g
MIGHTY KIDS MEALS				
Double Cheeseburger, Fries & Milk	810	40	16	79
Double Hamburger, Fries & Milk	700	31	11	78
McNuggets (6), Fries & Milk	570	28	8	56
SALADS				
California Cobb				
w/ Grilled Chicken	270	11	5	9
w/ Crispy Chicken	370	21	6	20
w/o Chicken	150	9	5	7
Chicken Bacon Ranch				
w/ Grilled Chicken	250	10	5	9
w/ Crispy Chicken	350	19	6	20
w/o Chicken	130	8	4	7
Chicken Caesar				
w/ Grilled Chicken	200	6	3	9
w/ Crispy Chicken	310	16	5	20
w/o Chicken	90	4	3	7
Fiesta	360	22	10	19
Side Salad	15	0	0	3
DRESSINGS & CONDIMENTS				
Cobb Dressing	120	9	2	9
Creamy Caesar Dressing	190	18	4	4
Low Fat Balsamic Vinaigrette	40	3	0	4
Ranch Dressing	170	15	3	9
Salsa	30	0	0	7
Sour Cream	60	5	3	2
BREAKFAST				
Bacon, Egg & Cheese McGriddle	440	21	7	43
Bacon, Egg & Cheese Biscuit	430	26	8	31
Bagel	260	1	0	54
Big Breakfast	700	47	13	45
Biscuit	240	11	3	30
Deluxe Breakfast	1190	61	15	130
Deluxe Warm Cinnamon Roll	510	23	8	81

	Calories	Fat g	Sat. Fat g	Carb. g
Egg McMuffin	300	12	5	29
Eggs, Scrambled (2)	160	11	4	1
English Muffin	150	2	1	27
Ham, Egg & Cheese Bagel	550	23	8	58
Hash Browns	130	8	2	14
Hotcakes (3)	340	8	2	58
Margarine (2 pats) & Syrup	260	17	1	46
Hotcakes & Sausage	780	33	9	104
Sausage	170	16	5	0
Biscuit	410	28	8	30
Breakfast Burrito	290	16	6	24
McGriddle	420	23	7	42
McMuffin	370	23	9	28
Biscuit w/ Egg	490	33	10	31
McMuffin w/ Egg	450	28	10	29
Egg & Cheese McGriddle	550	33	11	43
Spanish Omelete Bagel	710	40	15	59
Steak, Egg & Cheese Bagel	640	31	12	57
Warm Cinnamon Roll	440	19	5	60

DESSERTS

	Calories	Fat g	Sat. Fat g	Carb. g
Apple Dippers	35	0	0	8
w/ Low-Fat Caramel Dip	100	1	1	22
Baked Apple Pie	260	13	4	34
Chocolate Chip Cookie	160	8	2	22
Fruit 'n Yogurt Parfait	160	2	1	30
w/o Granola	130	2	1	25
Hot Caramel Sundae	360	10	6	61
Hot Fudge Sundae	340	12	9	52
Kiddie Cone	45	2	1	7
Low-Fat Caramel Dip	70	1	1	14
M&M McFlurry (12 fl oz)	630	23	15	90
McDonaldland Chocolate Chip Cookies	280	14	8	37
McDonaldland Cookies	230	8	2	38
Nuts for Sundaes	40	4	0	2
Oatmeal Raisin Cookie	150	6	1	23
Oreo McFlurry (12 fl oz)	570	20	12	82
Strawberry Sundae	290	7	5	50

	Calories	Fat g	Sat. Fat g	Carb. g
Sugar Cookie	140	6	1	20
Vanilla Reduced Fat Ice Cream Cone	150	5	3	23

MILKSHAKES, All Flavors

	Calories	Fat g	Sat. Fat g	Carb. g
Triple Thick Shake				
Chocolate				
12 fl oz	430	12	8	70
16 fl oz	580	17	11	94
21 fl oz	750	22	14	123
32 fl oz	1150	33	22	187
Strawberry				
12 fl oz	420	12	8	67
16 fl oz	560	16	11	89
21 fl oz	730	21	14	116
32 fl oz	1120	32	22	178
Vanilla				
12 fl oz	430	12	8	67
16 fl oz	570	16	11	89
21 fl oz	750	21	14	116
32 fl oz	1140	32	22	178

Values are subject to change; however, at the time of printing these were the values published at www.mcdonalds.com (6/4/04).

PANDA EXPRESS

	Calories	Fat g	Sat. Fat g	Carb. g
ENTRÉES				
BBQ Pork	350	19	7	13
Beef & Broccoli	150	8	2	9
Beef w/ String Beans	170	9	2	11
Black Pepper Chicken	180	10	2	10
Chicken w/ Pesto	220	11	2	17
Chicken with Mushrooms	130	7	2	7
Chicken with String Beans	170	8	2	12
Mandarin Chicken	250	9	3	8
Orange Chicken	480	21	5	50
Spicy Chicken with Peanuts	200	7	2	17
Sweet & Sour Chicken	310	14	3	28
Sweet & Sour Pork	410	30	7	17
SIDE ORDERS				
Chicken Egg Roll	190	8	2	21
Fried Shrimp	260	12	3	26
Mixed Vegetables	70	3	1	8
Steamed Rice	330	1	0	74
String Beans w/ Fried Tofu	180	11	2	11
Vegetable Chow Mein	330	11	2	48
Vegetable Fried Rice	390	12	3	61
Veggie Spring Roll	80	3	0	14
SAUCES				
Hot Mustard Sauce	18	0	0	1
Hot Sauce	10	1	0	2
Mandarin Sauce	70	0	0	16
Soy Sauce	16	0	0	3
Sweet & Sour Sauce	60	0	0	15

Values are subject to change; however, at the time of printing these were the values published at www.pandaexpress.com (10/4/04).

PIZZA HUT

	Calories	Fat g	Sat. Fat g	Carb. g
FIT 'N DELICIOUS MEDIUM (1 slice)				
Diced Chicken, Mushroom & Jalapeño	170	5	2	22
Diced Chicken, Red Onion & Green Pepper	170	5	2	23
Green Peppers, Red Onion & Diced Red Tomato	150	4	2	24
Ham, Pineapple and Diced Red Tomato	160	4	2	24
Ham, Red Onion & Mushroom	160	5	2	22
Tomato, Mushroom & Jalapeño	150	4	3	22
FIT 'N DELICIOUS LARGE (1 slice)				
Diced Chicken, Mushroom & Jalapeño	160	5	2	20
Diced Chicken, Red Onion & Green Pepper	160	4	2	22
HAND-TOSSED MEDIUM (1 slice)				
Cheese	240	8	5	30
Chicken Supreme	230	6	3	30
Ham	220	5	3	29
Meat Lover's	300	13	6	29
Pepperoni	250	9	5	29
Pepperoni Lover's	300	13	7	30
Sausage Lover's	280	12	5	30
Super Supreme	300	13	6	31
Supreme	270	11	5	30
Veggie Lover's	220	6	3	31
HAND-TOSSED LARGE (1 slice)				
Cheese	220	8	5	27
Chicken Supreme	210	6	3	28
Ham	200	6	3	27
Meat Lover's	280	12	5	27
Pepperoni	230	9	5	27
Pepperoni Lover's	280	13	6	27

	Calories	Fat g	Sat. Fat g	Carb. g
Sausage Lover's	260	11	5	27
Super Supreme	270	12	5	28
Supreme	250	10	5	28
Veggie Lover's	200	6	3	28

THIN 'N CRISPY MEDIUM (1 slice)

Cheese	200	8	5	21
Chicken Supreme	200	7	4	22
Ham	180	6	3	21
Meat Lover's	270	14	6	21
Pepperoni	210	10	5	21
Pepperoni Lover's	260	14	7	21
Super Supreme	260	13	6	23
Supreme	240	11	5	22
Veggie Lover's	180	7	3	23

THIN 'N CRISPY LARGE (1 slice)

Cheese	190	8	5	20
Chicken Supreme	180	6	3	21
Ham	170	6	3	19
Meat Lover's	250	13	6	20
Pepperoni	200	9	5	19
Pepperoni Lover's	250	14	5	20
Sausage Lover's	230	12	5	20
Super Supreme	240	12	5	21
Supreme	220	11	5	21
Veggie Lover's	170	7	3	21

PAN MEDIUM (1 slice)

Cheese	280	13	5	28
Chicken Supreme	280	12	4	30
Ham	260	11	4	29
Meat Lover's	340	19	7	29
Pepperoni	290	15	5	29
Pepperoni Lover's	340	19	7	29
Sausage Lover's	330	17	6	29
Super Supreme	340	18	6	30
Supreme	320	16	6	30
Veggie Lover's	260	12	4	30

	Calories	Fat g	Sat. Fat g	Carb. g
PAN LARGE (1 slice)				
Cheese	270	13	5	27
Chicken Supreme	260	11	4	27
Ham	250	11	4	26
Meat Lover's	320	18	6	27
Pepperoni	280	14	5	26
Pepperoni Lover's	330	18	7	27
Sausage Lover's	300	17	6	27
Super Supreme	320	17	6	28
Supreme	300	15	6	27
Veggie Lover's	250	11	4	28
6″ PERSONAL PAN (1 slice)				
Cheese	160	7	3	18
Chicken Supreme	160	6	3	19
Ham	150	6	2	18
Meat Lover's	200	10	4	18
Pepperoni	170	8	3	18
Pepperoni Lover's	200	10	5	18
Sausage Lover's	190	10	4	18
Super Supreme	200	16	4	19
Supreme	190	9	4	18
Veggie Lover's	150	6	2	18
STUFFED CRUST LARGE (1 slice)				
Cheese	360	13	8	43
Chicken Supreme	380	13	7	44
Meat Lover's	450	21	10	44
Pepperoni	370	15	8	42
Pepperoni Lover's	420	19	10	43
Sausage Lover's	430	19	9	43
Super Supreme	440	20	9	45
Supreme	400	16	8	44
Veggie Lover's	350	14	7	45
EXTRA LARGE (1 slice)				
Cheese	420	15	8	51
Chicken Supreme	400	12	6	52
Ham	380	12	6	50
Meat Lover's	500	22	10	51

	Calories	Fat g	Sat. Fat g	Carb. g
Pepperoni	430	17	8	50
Pepperoni Lover's	500	22	10	51
Sausage Lover's	510	23	10	51
Super Supreme	490	21	9	53
Supreme	460	19	9	52
Veggie Lover's	390	12	6	53
P'ZONES (1/2)				
Classic	610	21	11	71
Meat Lover's	680	28	14	70
Pepperoni	610	22	11	69
WINGS				
Hot Wings (2)	110	6	2	1
Mild Wings (2)	110	7	2	0
BREADSTICKS				
Breadstick (1)	150	6	1	20
Breadstick Dipping Sauce	50	0	0	11
Cheese Breadstick (1)	200	10	4	21
SAUCES				
Marinara Sauce	45	0	0	15
Wing Blue Cheese Dipping Sauce	230	24	5	2
Wing Ranch Dipping Sauce	210	22	4	4
DESSERTS				
Apple Dessert Pizza (1 slice)	260	4	1	53
Cherry Dessert Pizza (1 slice)	240	4	1	47
Cinnamon Sticks (2)	170	5	1	27
White Icing Dipping Cup (2 oz)	190	0	0	46

Values are subject to change; however, at the time of printing these were the values published at www.pizzahut.com (5/4/04).

SMOOTHIE KING

	Calories	Fat g	Sat. Fat g	Carb. g
LOW-FAT NUTRITIONAL SMOOTHIES (20 oz)				
Angel Food	330	1	0	79
Blackberry Dream	343	0	0	86
Blueberry Heaven	260	1	0	58
Caribbean Way	392	0	0	96
Celestial Cherry High	285	0	0	69
Cherry Picker	360	1	0	98
Cranberry Cooler	538	0	0	132
Cranberry Supreme	577	1	0	139
Grape Expectations	399	0	0	96
Grape Expectations Part II	529	0	0	129
Hearty Apple	380	2	1	81
Immune Builder	333	1	0	80
Instant Vigor	359	1	0	87
Island Treat	334	1	0	81
Lemon Twist Banana	339	0	0	82
Lemon Twist Strawberry	399	0	0	97
Light & Fluffy	389	0	0	98
Mangofest	320	0	0	78
Muscle Punch	339	1	0	80
Muscle Punch Plus	340	1	0	80
Orange Ka-BAM	320	0	0	104
Peach Slice	341	0	0	80
Peach Slice Plus	471	0	0	113
Pep Upper	334	0	0	80
Pineapple Pleasure	331	0	0	76
Pineapple Surf	440	1	0	104
Raspberry Sunrise	335	1	0	85
Slim-'N-Trim				
Chocolate	270	2	1	55
Orange Vanilla	199	0	0	43
Strawberry	357	1	0	79
Vanilla	227	1	0	51
Strawberry Kiwi Breeze	300	0	0	70
Strawberry X-Treme	370	0	0	91
Youth Fountain	267	0	0	65
WORKOUT SMOOTHIES (20 oz)				
Activator				
Chocolate	429	1	0	90
Strawberry	559	1	0	123
Vanilla	429	1	0	90

	Calories	Fat g	Sat. Fat g	Carb. g
Power Punch	430	1	0	102
Power Punch Plus	499	2	0	113
Super Punch	425	0	0	95
Super Punch Plus	516	0	0	118

WEIGHT GAIN SMOOTHIES (20 oz)
Hulk				
Chocolate	846	29	17	129
Strawberry	953	29	16	156
Vanilla	846	29	16	129
Malt	887	41	26	119
Peanut Power	502	21	4	72
Peanut Power Plus				
Grape	703	21	4	119
Strawberry	632	21	4	104
Shake	875	41	25	117

LOW-CARB SMOOTHIES (20 oz)
Banana	225	6	3	4
Chocolate	225	6	3	4
Strawberry	225	6	3	4
Vanilla	225	6	3	4

HIGH-PROTEIN SMOOTHIES (20 oz)
Almond Mocha	402	13	2	45
Banana	412	14	2	44
Chocolate	401	13	2	45
Lemon	390	13	2	41
Pineapple	380	13	2	41

SPECIALTY SMOOTHIES (20 oz)
Banana Boat	520	14	8	93
Coconut Surprise	457	6	2	99
Mo'cuccino	420	12	7	71
Piña Colada Island	550	11	9	102
Yogurt D-Lite	335	4	2	58

KID'S KUP SMOOTHIES (12 oz)
Berry Interesting	150	0	0	37
Choc-A-Laka	210	2	0	44
Gimme-Grape	170	0	0	42
Smarti Tarti	150	0	0	36

Values are subject to change; however, at the time of printing these were the values published at www.smoothieking.com (8/04).

STARBUCKS

	Calories	Fat g	Sat. Fat g	Carb. g
FRAPPUCCINO BLENDED COFFEE (Grande, 16 oz)				
Caffè Vanilla Frappuccino	340	4	2	72
w/ Whip	470	16	10	74
Caramel Frappuccino	280	4	2	57
w/ Whip	430	16	10	61
Coffee Frappuccino	260	4	2	52
Espresso Frappuccino	230	3	2	46
Java Chip Frappuccino	370	9	6	69
w/ Whip	510	22	15	73
Mocha Frappuccino	290	4	2	58
w/ Whip	420	16	10	61
Peppermint Mocha Frappuccino	310	4	2	63
w/ Whip	440	16	10	66
Pumpkin Spice Frappuccino	300	4	2	61
w/ Whip	430	16	10	63
Toffee Nut Frappuccino	280	4	2	58
w/ Whip	420	16	10	62
White Chocolate Mocha Frappuccino	320	5	3	62
w/ Whip	450	17	11	65
FRAPPUCCINO LIGHT BLENDED COFFEE (Grande, 16 oz)				
Caffè Vanilla Frappuccino Light	230	1	0	49
w/ Whip	360	13	8	51
Caramel Frappuccino Light	180	2	0	36
w/ Whip	310	14	8	39
Coffee Frappuccino Light	150	1	0	30
w/ Whip	280	13	8	32
Espresso Frappuccino Light	140	1	0	27
w/ Whip	270	13	8	29
Java Chip Frappuccino Light	260	7	5	46
w/ Whip	400	19	13	50
Mocha Frappuccino Light	180	2	0	36
w/ Whip	310	14	8	38
Pumpkin Spice Frappuccino Light	190	1	0	38
w/ Whip	320	13	8	41

	Calories	Fat g	Sat. Fat g	Carb. g
White Chocolate Mocha				
Frappuccino Light	200	3	1	40
w/ Whip	340	15	9	42

FRAPPUCCINO BLENDED CRÈME (Grande, 16 oz)

	Calories	Fat g	Sat. Fat g	Carb. g
Double Chocolate Chip				
Frappuccino Blended Crème	460	12	6	79
w/ Whip	590	24	14	83
Strawberries & Crème				
Frappuccino Blended Crème	450	5	2	90
w/ Whip	580	17	10	92
Tazo Chai Crème				
Frappuccino Blended Tea	380	5	2	72
w/ Whip	510	17	10	74
Toffee Nut Frappuccino Crème	360	5	1	65
w/ Whip	490	17	9	69
Vanilla Bean Frappuccino				
Blended Crème	370	5	2	70
w/ Whip	500	17	10	72

ESPRESSO-HOT (Grande, 16 oz)

	Calories	Fat g	Sat. Fat g	Carb. g
Café Misto (Café Au Lait)				
w/ Nonfat Milk	90	0	0	13
w/ Whole Milk	140	8	5	11
Breve	300	26	16	11
Caffè Latte				
w/ Nonfat Milk	160	0	0	24
w/ Whole Milk	260	14	9	21
Breve	550	47	29	20
Caffè Mocha				
w/ Nonfat Milk	230	2	0	43
w/ Whole Milk	300	12	7	41
Breve	510	37	22	40
w/ Nonfat Milk w/ Whip	330	12	7	44
w/ Whole Milk w/ Whip	400	22	13	42
Breve w/ Whip	610	46	28	41
Cappuccino				
w/ Nonfat Milk	100	0	0	14
w/ Whole Milk	150	8	5	13
Breve	310	27	17	12

	Calories	Fat g	Sat. Fat g	Carb. g
Caramel Macchiato				
w/ Nonfat Milk	220	1	1	40
w/ Whole Milk	310	12	7	37
Breve	550	41	26	36
Caramel Mocha				
w/ Nonfat Milk	300	3	0	63
w/ Whole Milk	370	11	6	61
Breve	560	34	20	60
w/ Nonfat Milk w/ Whip	410	12	7	65
w/ Whole Milk w/ Whip	470	21	12	63
Breve w/ Whip	660	43	26	62
Gingerbread Latte				
w/ Nonfat Milk	240	0	0	43
w/ Whole Milk	330	13	8	41
Breve	590	43	27	39
w/ Nonfat Milk w/ Whip	340	9	6	45
w/ Whole Milk w/ Whip	430	22	14	43
Breve w/ Whip	690	53	33	41
Pumpkin Spice Latte				
w/ Nonfat Milk	290	0	0	54
w/ Whole Milk	380	12	8	52
Breve	620	42	26	50
w/ Nonfat Milk w/ Whip	390	10	6	56
w/ Whole Milk w/ Whip	480	22	14	53
Breve w/ Whip	720	51	32	52
Syrup Flavored Latte				
w/ Nonfat Milk	200	0	0	38
w/ Whole Milk	280	10	6	36
Breve	490	35	22	35
Toffee Nut Latte				
w/ Nonfat Milk	230	0	0	43
w/ Whole Milk	330	13	8	41
Breve	580	43	27	39
w/ Nonfat Milk w/ Whip	340	10	6	47
w/ Whole Milk w/ Whip	430	22	14	44
Breve w/ Whip	690	53	33	43
Vanilla Latte				
w/ Nonfat Milk	200	0	0	38
w/ Whole Milk	280	10	6	36
Breve	490	35	22	35

	Calories	Fat g	Sat. Fat g	Carb. g
White Chocolate Mocha				
w/ Nonfat Milk	340	5	4	58
w/ Whole Milk	410	15	10	56
Breve	620	40	25	55
w/ Nonfat Milk w/ Whip	440	14	10	60
w/ Whole Milk w/ Whip	510	24	16	58
Breve w/ Whip	720	49	32	57
ESPRESSO-ICED (Grande, 16 oz)				
Iced Caffè Latte				
w/ Nonfat Milk	100	0	0	14
w/ Whole Milk	160	8	5	13
Iced Caffè Mocha				
w/ Nonfat Milk	180	2	0	36
w/ Whole Milk	220	8	4	35
w/ Nonfat Milk w/ Whip	310	14	9	38
w/ Whole Milk w/ Whip	350	20	12	37
Iced Caramel Macchiato				
w/ Nonfat Milk	200	1	1	36
w/ Whole Milk	270	10	6	34
Iced Syrup Flavored Latte				
w/ Nonfat Milk	160	0	0	32
w/ Whole Milk	210	7	4	31
Breve	360	24	15	30
Iced Vanilla Latte				
w/ Nonfat Milk	160	0	0	32
w/ Whole Milk	210	7	4	31
Breve	360	24	15	30
Iced White Chocolate Mocha				
w/ Nonfat Milk	320	6	5	57
w/ Whole Milk	360	11	8	56
w/ Nonfat Milk w/ Whip	450	18	12	59
w/ Whole Milk w/ Whip	490	24	16	58
TAZO TEA (Grande, 16 oz)				
Iced Tazo Chai Tea Latte				
w/ Nonfat Milk	230	0	0	50
w/ Whole Milk	270	7	4	48

	Calories	Fat g	Sat. Fat g	Carb. g
Tazo Chai Tea Latte				
w/ Nonfat Milk	230	0	0	51
w/ Whole Milk	290	7	5	50
Breve	430	25	15	49
Tazo Iced Tea	80	0	0	21
Tazo Tea Lemonade	120	0	0	30
			4	

CLASSIC FAVORITES (Grande, 16 oz)

	Calories	Fat g	Sat. Fat g	Carb. g
Caramel Apple Cider	300	0	0	72
w/ Whip	410	10	7	76
Chocolate Milk				
w/ Nonfat Milk	240	2	0	45
w/ Whole Milk	340	15	8	42
Breve	600	46	28	41
Hot Chocolate				
w/ Nonfat Milk	240	2	0	45
w/ Whole Milk	340	15	8	42
Breve	600	46	28	41
w/ Nonfat Milk w/ Whip	340	12	7	47
w/ Whole Milk w/ Whip	440	24	15	44
Breve w/ Whip	700	55	34	43
Toffee Nut Crème				
w/ Nonfat Milk	250	0	0	44
w/ Whole Milk	350	15	9	41
Breve	650	50	31	40
w/ Nonfat Milk w/ Whip	350	10	6	48
w/ Whole Milk w/ Whip	460	24	15	45
Breve w/ Whip	760	60	37	43
Vanilla Crème				
w/ Nonfat Milk	230	0	0	43
w/ Whole Milk	330	14	8	39
Breve	630	49	30	38
w/ Nonfat Milk w/ Whip	330	9	6	44
w/ Whole Milk w/ Whip	440	23	14	41
Breve w/ Whip	730	58	37	40

	Calories	Fat g	Sat. Fat g	Carb. g
White Hot Chocolate				
w/ Nonfat Milk	390	6	5	66
w/ Whole Milk	480	18	12	63
Breve	740	49	32	62
w/ Nonfat Milk w/ Whip	490	15	11	68
w/ Whole Milk w/ Whip	580	28	19	65
Breve w/ Whip	840	59	38	64

Values are subject to change; however, at the time of printing these were the values published at www.starbucks.com (11/8/04).

SUBWAY

	Calories	Fat g	Sat. Fat g	Carb. g
6" SUB SANDWICHES				
Baja Chicken	350	9	2	45
Baja Pork	530	21	7	50
Barbecue Pulled Pork	440	13	5	53
BBQ Rib Patty	420	19	7	47
Buffalo Chicken	400	15	4	45
Carne Asada	420	11	1	45
Cheese Steak	360	10	5	47
Chicken Fajita	510	21	8	49
Chipotle Southwest Cheese Steak	440	19	6	49
Classic Tuna	430	19	5	46
Cold Cut Combo	410	17	7	46
Dijon Turkey Breast, Ham & Bacon Melt	470	21	7	48
Double Meat				
Cheese Steak	450	14	6	50
Chicken	430	8	3	50
Chipotle Southwest Cheese Steak	530	22	7	52
Classic Tuna	580	32	7	48
Cold Cut Combo	550	28	10	48
Italian BMT	630	35	14	49
Ham	350	7	3	49
Meatball Marinara	740	38	18	61
Roast Beef	360	7	4	46
Seafood Sensation	490	20	5	60
Sweet Onion Chicken Teriyaki	450	7	2	59
Turkey Breast & Ham	360	7	2	48
Turkey Breast	330	5	2	48
Turkey Breast, Ham & Bacon Melt	490	17	8	51
Turkey Breast, Ham & Roast Beef	410	8	3	49
Gardenburger	390	7	3	66
Ham	290	5	2	46
Honey Mustard Ham	310	5	2	54
Italian BMT	450	21	8	47

	Calories	Fat g	Sat. Fat g	Carb. g
Lloyd's BBQ Chicken	310	6	2	52
Meatball Marinara	500	22	11	52
Mediterranean Chicken	440	16	6	48
Oven Roasted Chicken Breast	330	5	2	47
Pastrami	570	29	9	49
Roast Beef	290	5	2	45
Savory Chicken Caesar	490	23	6	46
Savory Turkey Breast & Ham	290	5	2	46
Savory Turkey Breast	280	5	2	46
Spicy Italian	480	25	9	45
Steak Fajita	500	21	8	52
Subway Seafood Sensation	380	13	5	52
Sweet Onion Chicken Teriyaki	370	5	2	59
Turkey Breast				
w/ Ham & Bacon Melt	380	12	5	47
w/ Ham & Roast Beef	320	6	2	47
Veggie Delite	230	3	1	44
Veggi-Max	390	8	2	56

DELI SANDWICHES

	Calories	Fat g	Sat. Fat g	Carb. g
Classic Tuna	300	13	5	36
Ham	210	4	2	35
Roast Beef	220	5	2	35
Savory Turkey Breast	210	4	2	36

WRAPS

	Calories	Fat g	Sat. Fat g	Carb. g
Chicken Bacon Ranch	440	26	9	17
Turkey Bacon Melt	430	27	10	20
Turkey Breast & Ham	390	23	8	19

SALADS

	Calories	Fat g	Sat. Fat g	Carb. g
Classic Club	390	21	10	13
Garden Fresh	60	1	0	11
Grilled Chicken & Spinach	420	26	10	10
Mediterranean Chicken	170	5	2	11

SALAD DRESSINGS

	Calories	Fat g	Sat. Fat g	Carb. g
Fat Free Italian	35	0	0	7
Ranch	200	22	4	1
Red Wine Vinaigrette	80	1	0	17

	Calories	Fat g	Sat. Fat g	Carb. g
CONDIMENTS				
Bacon Bits	60	5	2	0
Chipotle Southwest Sauce	90	9	2	2
Croutons	30	0	0	8
Diced Eggs	30	3	1	0
Dijon Horseradish Sauce	90	10	2	1
Fat Free Honey Mustard Sauce	30	0	0	7
Fat Free Red Wine Vinaigrette Sauce	30	0	0	6
Fat Free Sweet Onion Sauce	40	0	0	9
Garlic Almonds	80	7	1	3
Olive Oil Blend	45	5	1	0
BREAKFAST				
Bacon & Egg				
Omelet	240	17	6	2
Sandwich	320	15	5	34
Sub	450	19	7	42
Cheese & Egg				
Omelet	240	17	6	2
Sandwich	320	15	5	34
Sub	440	19	7	42
French Toast w/ Syrup	350	8	3	57
Ham & Egg				
Omelet	230	14	5	2
Sandwich	310	13	4	34
Sub	430	17	5	42
Steak & Egg				
Omelet	250	15	5	3
Sandwich	330	14	4	35
Sub	460	18	6	43
Vegetable & Egg				
Omelet	210	14	4	4
Sandwich	290	12	3	36
Sub	410	16	5	44
Western & Egg				
Omelet	220	14	5	4
Sandwich	300	12	4	36
Sub	430	17	5	44

	Calories	Fat g	Sat. Fat g	Carb. g
DESSERTS				
Apple Pie	245	10	2	37
Chocolate Chip Cookie	210	10	4	30
Chocolate Chunk Cookie	220	10	4	30
Double Chocolate Chip Cookie	210	10	4	30
Fruit Roll Up	50	1	0	12
M&M Cookie	210	10	4	30
Oatmeal Raisin Cookie	200	8	3	30
Peanut Butter Cookie	220	12	4	26
Sugar Cookie	230	12	4	28
White Macadamia Nut Cookie	220	11	4	28
BEVERAGES				
Fruizle Express				
Berry Lishus	110	0	0	28
Berry Lishus w/ Banana	140	0	0	35
Peach Pizazz	100	0	0	26
Pineapple Delight	130	0	0	33
w/ Banana	160	0	0	40
Sunrise Refresher	120	0	0	29

Values are subject to change; however, at the time of printing these were the values published at www.subway.com (5/4/04).

TACO BELL

	Calories	Fat g	Sat. Fat g	Carb. g

Any item with cheese and/or sauce can be made Fresco Style (salsa replaces cheese and/or sauce).

TACOS

	Calories	Fat g	Sat. Fat g	Carb. g
Double Decker Taco	340	14	5	39
Double Decker Taco Supreme	380	18	8	40
Fresco Style Soft Taco				
Beef	190	8	3	22
Chicken	170	4	1	20
Grilled Steak	170	4	2	21
Ranchero Chicken	170	4	1	22
Fresco Style Crunchy Taco	150	7	3	14
Soft Taco Supreme				
Beef	260	14	7	22
Chicken	230	10	5	21
Soft Taco				
Beef	210	10	5	21
Chicken	190	6	3	19
Grilled Steak	280	17	5	21
Taco	170	10	4	13
Taco Supreme	220	14	7	14

GORDITAS

	Calories	Fat g	Sat. Fat g	Carb. g
Fresco Style Gordita Baja				
Beef	250	9	3	30
Chicken	230	6	1	29
Steak	230	7	2	29
Gordita Baja				
Beef	350	19	5	31
Chicken	320	15	4	29
Steak	320	16	4	29
Gordita Nacho Cheese				
Beef	300	13	4	32
Chicken	270	10	3	30
Steak	270	11	3	30
Gordita Supreme				
Beef	310	16	7	30
Chicken	290	12	5	28
Steak	290	13	6	28

	Calories	Fat g	Sat. Fat g	Carb. g
BURRITOS				
7-Layer Burrito	530	22	8	67
Bean Burrito	370	10	4	55
Burrito Supreme				
Beef	440	18	8	51
Chicken	410	14	6	50
Steak	420	16	7	50
Chili Cheese Burrito	390	18	9	40
Fiesta Burrito				
Beef	390	15	5	50
Chicken	370	12	4	48
Steak	370	13	4	48
Fresco Style Bean Burrito	350	8	2	56
Fresco Style Burrito Supreme				
Chicken	350	8	2	50
Steak	350	9	3	50
Fresco Style Fiesta Burrito,				
Chicken	350	9	2	49
Grilled Stuft Burrito				
Beef	730	33	11	79
Chicken	680	26	7	76
Steak	680	28	8	76
CHALUPAS				
Chalupa Baja				
Beef	430	27	8	32
Chicken	400	24	6	30
Steak	400	25	7	30
Chalupa Nacho Cheese				
Beef	380	22	7	33
Chicken	350	18	5	31
Steak	350	19	5	31
Chalupa Supreme				
Beef	390	24	10	31
Chicken	370	20	8	30
Steak	370	22	8	29
TOSTADAS				
Fresco Style Tostada	200	6	1	30
Tostada	250	10	4	29

	Calories	Fat g	Sat. Fat g	Carb. g
ENCHIRITOS				
Enchirito				
Beef	380	18	9	35
Chicken	350	14	7	33
Steak	360	16	8	33
Fresco Style Enchirito				
Beef	270	9	3	35
Chicken	250	5	2	34
Steak	250	7	2	34
QUESADILLAS				
Cheese	490	28	13	39
Chicken	540	30	13	40
Steak	540	31	14	40
NACHOS				
Nachos	320	19	5	33
BellGrande	780	43	13	80
Supreme	450	26	9	42
SPECIALTIES				
Mexican Pizza	550	31	11	46
MexiMelt	290	16	8	23
SALADS				
Express Taco Salad				
w/ Chips	620	31	13	60
Southwest Steak Bowl	700	32	8	73
Taco Salad				
w/ Salsa	790	42	15	73
w/ Salsa w/o Shell	420	21	11	33
Zesty Chicken Border Bowl				
w/ Dressing	730	42	9	65
w/o Dressing	500	19	5	60
SIDE ORDERS				
Mexican Rice	210	10	4	23
Pintos'n Cheese	180	7	4	20

	Calories	Fat g	Sat. Fat g	Carb. g
CONDIMENTS & DRESSINGS				
Border Sauce				
Fire	15	0	0	3
Hot	10	0	0	1
Mild	5	0	0	1
Cheddar Cheese	110	9	6	0
Creamy Jalapeño Sauce	140	14	3	3
Creamy Lime Sauce	180	19	3	2
Fiesta Salsa	5	0	0	2
Green Sauce	10	0	0	2
Guacamole	50	4	1	3
Nacho Cheese Sauce	35	4	1	3
Pepper Jack Cheese Sauce	150	15	3	2
Red Sauce	10	0	0	2
Sour Cream	60	5	4	1
Three-Cheese Blend	100	8	5	
Zesty Dressing	160	16	3	3
BREAKFAST				
Breakfast Burrito	510	25	9	48
Breakfast Gordita	380	24	7	28
Breakfast Quesadilla	400	20	9	38
Breakfast Steak Burrito	500	26	10	40
Breakfast Steak Quesadilla w/ Green Sauce	460	23	10	39
DESSERT				
Cinnamon Twists	160	5	1	28

Values are subject to change; however, at the time of printing these were the values published at www.tacobell.com (5/4/04).

CHAPTER 5

TRAVELING

AIRLINE AND CRUISE SHIP CUISINE

Most airlines offer snacks, beverages, and meals, and some airlines offer special meals. If special meals are available, those that are lowest in fat and saturated fat are "low-fat," "low-cholesterol," "low-calorie," and "diabetic." The best time to request a special meal is when you make your reservation.

For long airline flights, you may prefer to take your own food, such as nuts, crackers with peanut butter, fruit, low-fat cheese, or pretzels. A wide variety of beverages are available in flight, such as skim milk and fruit juices.

Passengers on cruise ships can choose from an abundance of food, often made available morning, noon, night, and in between. The dinner menu on a cruise ship typically offers a number of courses, including appetizer, soup, salad, pasta, main course, and dessert. Some cruise ship menus indicate foods that are low in cholesterol; these dishes may *not* be low in fat and/or saturated fat. It takes some planning and self-control to select reasonable amounts of foods that are lower in fat from among the numerous dishes being offered. The tips on selecting foods lower in fat that are listed throughout this book also apply to cruise ship cuisine.

JET LAG

Anyone who travels long distances by air may suffer the effects of jet lag. Jet lag may be recognized by fatigue, sleepiness, inability to sleep, gastrointestinal upset, and/or decreased mental alertness. It is a disturbance of the body's normal cycle of sleeping and waking—the biological clock—that is caused by flying across time zones.

Decreasing Jet Lag

- Sleep as much as possible on the airplane—ask that the flight attendant not awaken you for meals. Sleeping is much more important than reading, studying, or writing.
- Eat a light meal before boarding the airplane, since a heavy meal tends to increase fatigue and to interfere with sleep.
- During the flight, drink plenty of fluids that do not have caffeine or alcohol. To avoid dehydration, drink two 8-ounce glasses of water before a flight and one 12-ounce bottle of water for each hour of flight. Although some travelers think that alcohol has a tranquilizing effect, the ultimate result is increased fatigue and a depression of mental alertness.
- Assume the local schedule of eating and sleeping as soon as you reach your destination. Being outdoors in the sunlight helps you adjust to the new light–dark cycle.

GASTROINTESTINAL UPSET IN FOREIGN COUNTRIES

One of the pleasures of visiting foreign countires is the food of that culture. However, the water and certain foods can make you sick.

Decreasing the Risk for Gastrointestinal Upset in Foreign Countries

- Eat only foods that are cooked. Raw foods washed in the local water may carry bacteria that will cause diarrhea or nausea. Avoid all raw vegetables and fruits except fruits that can be peeled, such as bananas and oranges.
- Drink only bottled water with sealed cap and avoid ice. This includes the water used to take medications and to brush your teeth.
- Carbonated soft drinks, wine, beer, and other alcholic beverages are usually safe; however, the top of the container should be wiped with a antiseptic towelette before opening. Avoid putting cans or bottles to your mouth (use a straw).

- Avoid undercooked meat, which may contain parasites.
- Avoid meat held at room temperature for several hours because it allows bacteria to grow.
- Avoid ground meat, even if cooked.
- Avoid shelled nuts.
- Avoid acquatic, oriental plants such as watercress and water chestnuts.
- Avoid unpasteurized dairy products.

ABOUT THE AUTHORS

Michael E. DeBakey, M.D., pre-eminent cardiovascular surgeon, is internationally acclaimed as an ingenious medical inventor and innovator, a gifted and dedicated teacher, and a premier surgeon. Dr. DeBakey has served as President, Chairman of the Department of Surgery, and Chancellor of Baylor College of Medicine. He is now Chancellor Emeritus, Distinguished Service Professor and Olga Keith Wiess Professor of Surgery, in the Michael E. DeBakey Department of Surgery and Director of the DeBakey Heart Center, which was established by Baylor and The Methodist Hospital in 1985 for research and public education in the prevention and treatment of Heart Disease.

Dr. DeBakey performed the first successful coronary artery bypass, first successful carotid endarterectomy for stroke, the first excision and graft replacement for aneurysms of the descending, ascending thoracic aortas, and the aortic arch and for dissecting aneurysm. He also developed the first successful clinical application of Dacron® and Dacron®-velour graft for replacement of aneurysms and occlusive diseases of the aorta and major arteries. In 1966, he performed the first successful use of a left ventricular bypass pump for heart failure.

Because of his unique ability to bring his professional knowledge to bear on public policy worldwide, Dr. DeBakey is known as an international medical statesman. He has served as advisor to virtually every United States President in the past fifty years and to heads-of-state throughout the world. He has received 60 honorary degrees from prestigious colleges and universities, as well as innumerable awards from educational institutions, professional and civic organizations, and governments worldwide. These include the prestigious Lasker Award, the U.S. Army Legion of Merit Award, the Rudolph Matas Award in Vascular Surgery, the Presidential Medal of Freedom with Distinction, the National Medal of Science, and the Library of Congress Living Legend Award.

Dr. DeBakey's lifelong scholarship is reflected in more than 1600 published medical articles, chapters, and books on various aspects of surgery, medicine, health, medical research, and medical education, as well as related ethical, socioeconomic, and philosophic issues. In addition, he is a co-author of *The Living Heart* series of popular books for the public, a layman's guide to the heart and heart disease, including *The Living Heart* (1977), *The Living Heart Brand Name Shopper's Guide* (1993), *The Living Heart Guide to Eating Out* (1993), and *The New Living Heart* (1997), which was on The New York Times Best Seller list.

Dr. DeBakey's keen intellect, professional ingenuity, personal integrity, and selfless devotion in service to humanity have made him a legend in his own time.

Antonio M. Gotto, Jr., M.D., D.Phil., is the Stephen and Suzanne Weiss Dean of Weill Medical College of Cornell University, New York City, New York, where he is also a Professor of Medicine. He is also the Provost for Medical Affairs for Cornell University. Previously, he spent over two decades at Baylor College of Medicine in Houston, Texas, where he was the Bob and Vivian Smith Professor and Chairman of the Albert B. and Margaret M. Alkek Department of Medicine and the Chief of the Internal Medicine Service at The Methodist Hospital in Houston, Texas. During that time, he also held the J. S. Abercrombie Professor Chair for Atherosclerosis and Lipoprotein Research and was the Scientific Director of The DeBakey Heart Center at Baylor.

Dr. Gotto has served as National President of the American Heart Association, as a member of the National Heart, Lung, and Blood Advisory Council, and on the National Diabetes Advisory Board. He is a member of the Institute of Medicine and of the American Academy of Arts and Sciences. He was the recipient of the 2000 Distinguished Alumnus award from Vanderbilt University and the Vanderbilt University School of Medicine. He has received honorary doctoral degrees from the University of Bologna and Abilene Christian University and honorary professorships from the University of Buenos Aires and Francisco Marroquin University (Guatemala). He is a Past-President of the International Atherosclerosis Society and Co-Chairman of the US Russian and US Italian Cardiovascular Work groups. He has received the Order of the Lion from the Republic of Finland. Dr. Gotto is coauthor of *The New Living Heart*, and *The New Living Heart Diet*, which explain the origin and dietary treatment of cardiovascular disease to the general public; he is author of *The Living Heart Cookbook*. His original scholarly articles number well over 400.

Lynne W. Scott, M.A., R.D., L.D., is Assistant Professor in the Department of Medicine at Baylor College of Medicine. She is Director of the Diet Modification Clinic and Bionutritionist for the Adult General Clinical Research Center. She has served as a member of the National Cholesterol Education Program Expert Panel on Blood Cholesterol Levels in Children and Adolescents. She is a clinical researcher and conducts research investigating the effect of dietary components on lipids and lipoproteins. She developed the Internet Dietary Management System for helping patients make dietary changes. She is coauthor of *The Living Heart Diet*, which was on the New York Times Best Seller List, *The New Living Heart Diet, The Living Heart Guide To Eating Out,* and *The Living Heart Brand Name Shopper's Guide,* among about 50 publications.

ORDER FORM

Print Name _____

Address   _____

           _____

City _____ State ____ Zip _____

Please send me the book(s) indicated below:

_____ Copy(s) of THE LIVING HEART GUIDE TO
       EATING OUT at $11.95 each = $ _____

_____ Copy(s) of THE LIVING HEART BRAND NAME
       SHOPPER'S GUIDE at $14.95 each = $ _____

_____ Copy(s) of THE NEW LIVING HEART DIET
       at $16.00 each = $ _____

> Add $4.00 postage and handling for
> the first book and $1.50 for
> each additional book $_____
>
> Total enclosed $_____

Make payment by check or money order payable to Living Heart.

Please send to:
Living Heart
2001 Holcombe #2702
Houston, TX 77030

713-794-0240

Order Online at www.LivingHeart.com

ORDER FORM

Print Name _____

Address _____

_____

City _____ State ____ Zip _____

Please send me the book(s) indicated below:

____ Copy(s) of THE LIVING HEART GUIDE TO
EATING OUT at $11.95 each = $ _____

____ Copy(s) of THE LIVING HEART BRAND NAME
SHOPPER'S GUIDE at $14.95 each = $ _____

____ Copy(s) of THE NEW LIVING HEART DIET
at $16.00 each = $ _____

Add $4.00 postage and handling for
the first book and $1.50 for
each additional book $_____

Total enclosed $_____

Make payment by check or money order payable to Living Heart.

Please send to:
Living Heart
2001 Holcombe #2702
Houston, TX 77030

713-794-0240

Order Online at www.LivingHeart.com